LIV

WITHIN A

LIFE

Hope that this
enlighten you,
Thankyou for
your Support,

Rob

Robert Bayley

signing his book at
Daily Bread Cooporative
15/10/11

chipmunkapublishing
the mental health publisher
empowering people with schizophrenia

Robert Bayley

Published by
Chipmunkapublishing
PO Box 6872
Brentwood
Essex CM13 1ZT
United Kingdom

http://www.chipmunkapublishing.com

Chipmunkapublishing gratefully acknowledges the support of Arts Council England.

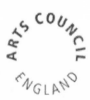

LIVES WITHIN A LIFE

PREFACE TO 'LIVES WITHIN A LIFE'

Novels by authors suffering from severe mental illness are a rarity. Diaries and factual accounts of the illness yes, but more imaginative writing requires a degree of detachment and self-control that is almost incompatible with a mind periodically overwhelmed by irrational thoughts and fears. Nowadays we are often told that great writers from the past such as Charles Dickens may have suffered from manic depression (or bipolar disorder to give it its more current name), but the fact is that nobody can offer an accurate diagnosis for someone they have never met – let alone treated – and it is questionable whether the condition of those writers would have satisfied to-day's diagnostic criteria.

Robert Bayley does not in any case fall into this category. I have known him for many years and admired his creativity and courage. He suffers from schizophrenia and his life is a constant struggle with its often mysterious manifestations: paranoid delusions, aggressive voices and intense anxiety. Yet Robert, through sheer force of will, has succeeded in writing a novel which draws on his own experience but which also transcends it, rising above the dark clouds in his head to touch a universal radiance. It is a story of one man's escape from the confines of his troubled life to a world redeemed by faith and love. It has been many years in the making and is by any standards a great achievement.

MARJORIE WALLACE - CHIEF EXECUTIVE OF SANE.

ALL AUTHOR PROFITS FROM THIS PUBLICATION WILL GO TO SUPPORT SANE, A CHARITY WHICH HELPS THOSE WITH SCHIZOPHRENIA AND OTHER SERIOUS MENTAL ILLNESS.

LIVES WITHIN A LIFE

ACKNOWLEDGEMENTS

Special thanks for making my work possible.

To my dearest wife, Gill, my wonderful Mother and Father and sisters, and my whole, extended family, for their constant compassion and support.

To David Gladstone for his invaluable input in helping to edit my book and to Marjorie Wallace for her encouragement.

To Jane Roberts, (BA Fine Art) for the cover photography, and Jeff Clark, (BA Fine Art) for design and promotion.

To all my fantastic friends for their loyalty and belief in me.

To Bill Simons and all at the Order of St.Luke for spiritual guidance.

To Julia Kingsford and Foyles Book Shop for their generous provision of their launch gallery.

To The Neighbours' Mental Health Trust for their kindness.

Finally, to the clinicians and specialists who have treated me over the years, especially Dr. Ferguson, Dr. Smart, and Dr. McCabe and his colleagues at The National Psychosis Unit.

Robert Bayley

LIVES WITHIN A LIFE

CONTENTS

Robert Bayley

LIVES WITHIN A LIFE

CHAPTER ONE - JON

The air was dry and the heatwave biting. The evergreens stood proud, resisting the scorching temperature. A mood of playfulness was captured by all. The youngest were left under the tranquil shelter of the weeping willows. Innocence encompassed those present, the sky streaked by an Impressionist's variegated palette, balloons ascending. An idyllic day to share and remember.

Five year old Jon was darting across the sea of green, his smile broad, as the other children shared his sense of fun. To the subdued tempo of the tender breeze, the trees swayed gently, their branches dancing, as the lake rippled in sympathy. The water reflected the shimmering light, the sun prickly on the skin. It was for all a time of whirling exultation. There were no concerns or cares, only a shared desire to absorb the beautiful surroundings. Sounds of festivity echoed with profundity, as Jon played with the shadows. He leapt from the foliage, immersed in laughter, as he lost himself to the world.

His parents looked on, as they chatted freely with friends and family. The wine flowed, accompanied by cheese and anecdotes. The birds above seemed to share the jollity and were full in song. Balls of all sizes cavorted across the turf as a group of players scrambled for a touch. There were screams of congratulations as each goal was scored. Ducks clambered onto the bank, devouring the crumbs of bread thrown for them. By the grass verge swans displayed their elegant splendour. The air became still, concentrating the heat, and creating demand for the chilled lemonade in the cooler. A spectrum of differing breeds of dog were bounding and barking across the slopes. Today was a wonderful day and by its close Jon was tired but still exuberant.

The heavens projected the softest of hues as the family left their place of delight, with no sense of foreboding. Surrounding them were fields of corn, their coloration intensified by rays above, forming perfectly symmetrical patterns.

Jon's heart had been cosseted by a magical experience, the sensations bold and true. Everything had become animated and inspired, the meandering line of the branches, the call of the wildlife, all contributing to a striking picture. Jon had floated with the balloons and never wanted to descend, for he had discovered life beyond the events of the day. Now he was earthbound, drenched in anticipation. The vibrancy was so overwhelming that Jon imagined each blade of grass suspended in isolation, and he gave thanks.

But this time of reflection led to a shooting forth. Minute organisms multiplied as Jon faced masks conveying a forever altering symbolism. As the night sky bombarded his soul, Jon was led into a place of confinement. The darkening mass was all enveloping as he longed to return to the sea of petals.

What a strange boy, he seems to possess a peculiar vision. He remains static for hours, transfixed upon a world only he can see. At times he becomes animated, the stimulus unknown. Youthful dreams spoke of fear and abstraction, perhaps a generation away, as though a loaded gun. At dawn Jon was free, by dusk he was ensnared. His head was erupting with nothing to contain it. Images fragmented, reason removed. For the demons had stormed the heart of a child so pure. The roar of spiritual collision was received, creating a deranged assemblage. What had occurred that fateful day when the boy returned with space in his eyes?

At school the next day expletives curled their ugly lip as Jon endeavoured to rise above the ominous behaviour that surrounded him. He clasped himself inside, and although his desk had previously been something of a haven, he now felt exposed and vulnerable.

The sun cast linear shadows across scarred and tarnished wooden beams, and the atmosphere in the classroom was oppressive. It had been a day of tedium, with little to preoccupy Jon.

Conversation in his classroom had veered towards matters unsavoury and Jon began to feel uneasy. His brow burned as Liz glared from across the desk. He was left feeling threatened. Liz's laughter was mocking and derisive as he vainly attempted to conceal his revulsion towards the content of her chatter. This abhorrence manifested itself by way of internal discord as Liz continued to use foul and disturbing language that shocked and repulsed Jon's sense of values.

Jon became gradually aware that a darkness had infiltrated the luminescence of a brighter day. Only an hour earlier he had been careering around the playground, seeing the world through a Disney cartoon viewer. Explosions of technicolor had flashed across the sky, with Pluto winking playfully and Donald Duck cavorting mischievously, provoking a feeling that tickled his senses. Today he knew a doorway had been opened, propelling him to fanciful extremes. Jon had contemplated the notion that he had also witnessed unearthly apparitions, something that he had not yet resolved.

What was definite was a passion for charged and intense imagery that launched him still further into a state of visual intoxication.

From this, Jon's attention had been diverted by Liz's harshness and crudity, leaving him distressed. He was concerned by the language she had used. It seemed to indicate a sense of darkness and malediction that felt like a stab deep into his flesh. But it was easier to conform and go with the flow and he gave in, weakly. As school drew to a close Jon felt wretched, his conscience troubled.

As his classmates filed through orderly classrooms, Jon's field of vision descended from the glistening peaks of the decorated schoolhouse to gargoyles enveloped by shadow and decay. They had a macabre, minatory air. The whole emphasis of the day had been transformed. The disturbances of the afternoon began to engulf Jon as he reflected upon the uneasy symbolism that had been projected upon him. The wall that during the day served as a goal for those children dynamic and playful, now appeared to confine Jon as sombre clouds formed above. He huddled in a corner, the schoolyard deserted.

By now Jon's innocent reality had become distorted, propelling him to extreme realms. Forms of a reptilian nature had infiltrated his psyche, edging in from the periphery of paranoid existence. Patterns in the tarmac appeared to proliferate, weaving a web of overwhelming complexity. As Jon trod a careful path towards the gates, he heard the faintest murmur from within. Although ill defined, it resonated deeply and began to shift in tonality, seemingly devoid of any sense of order. Appearing alien in their content, samples of sound formed linkages within, as an icy wind located his startled frame. Jon clasped his head, his cries futile, for a seed of despair had been sown. He gently rocked back and forth, wracked by confusion and disarray. Time stood still while a crow perched itself upon a rooftop and the surrounding stonework turned sepia as the light failed. Jon felt remorse when he recalled his reluctance to confront Liz's obdurate tongue. Was this a penalty for the weakness he had displayed previously?

The turbulent nature of events had left their mark by way of internal wounding, and now Jon was alone again. Almost without volition he rose to his feet, whilst concurrently a brilliant light appeared in the otherwise bleak sky. It was then that the day closed and he drifted into the night.

Jon's mother called him, exasperated by his apparent retreat. But he was lost in impressions of fragmented shapes that formed a film across his eyes. His mother's voice had faded, seeming indirect and distant. The need to connect dissipated as all perception was embedded in surrealism. To be conscious whilst dreaming, awake whilst yearning. The day when expletives dominated was to precipitate the commencement of demonic onslaught, and Jon was left shattered and alone. The ground beneath him was akin to a map of orderly veins, all parallels and angularities. Jon fell to his knees, only to find himself lost in another world.

Predators loomed large, the locality darkened. Jon wanted to play even though his eyes were streaming - where had everybody gone? That sense of loss, what could equate with it? The corridors revealed inner passages as Jon lay down, silent and contained by his experiences.

LIVES WITHIN A LIFE

As his mind reflected, Jon gazed from the window whilst pockets of steam emanated from the drains, only to disperse into elements severe. Outside, the cloudburst displayed its violence to all. Was this a fantastical world ready to reveal itself with wild abandonment?

The curtains were drawn, lights out. There was nothing, as far as the eye could see. But the perimeters had changed, objects inanimate coming to life, the toys in the cupboard taking charge.

Life was coming from a different angle, the waves colliding, the tongues whipping and cursing to a frenetic pitch. An arena of terror had evolved, Jon ventured, as the minutes turned into days into years.

Racing ahead towards new horizons, Jon could see origins of colour and form. When he was placed at a distance, he was able to recall events with great clarity. Whether treated with suspicion or otherwise, Jon felt compelled to inform, to enlighten. Was he evolving into an enigmatic figure, condemned by the wider world only for his observation?

Jon had begun to feel remote and challenged. Any sense of order was now diminishing. Whilst conceptualising, Jon would walk along the avenue towards home, breaking into a skip from time to time. To enjoy some richness of thought, however perceived. To meander, with autumn leaves crisp beneath each step. The road was bare, only a click of the heels to be heard. For brief moments, nothing seemed to register at all.

On the horizon there was much to be revealed, much to discover.

Some time had passed and Jon was travelling with his parents to visit his great aunt and her son. One of those trips of duty, precious when lost. He was at such a young age that maybe it would not make any impression. As to whether he was looking forward to the trip he was uncertain, as he was not familiar with these members of his extended family. His thoughts were more focused on the loss of an opportunity to play football with friends that same afternoon. He had been looking forward to the contact with his contemporaries, as he often existed on the fringe of his social grouping. As the car accelerated, edges of the road formed a blur, and Jon's attention was turned to the radiance of the mid-day sun and the clusters of clouds above. He took a photograph inside his head. Then it all went hazy, and before long he had drifted into a light sleep, only to be awoken by the sound of a heavy lorry as they approached their destination. Jon was initially disorientated but soon warmed to his first sight of the surrounding area.

As they entered the driveway, he was immediately struck by the vividness of the vast range of plants and flowers adorning the entrance to the house. Petals of deepest crimson and indigo framed the scene with beauty. Elegant trees led away from the patio, and the foliage was profuse. Jon gained the impression of a quaint, well cared for dwelling. It was the perfect scene for a watercolour with which to enhance a wall. The roof was elaborately thatched, the brickwork fashioned from crumbling stone. Jon was intrigued by its location, being set well apart from the other properties. There was much to absorb as the atmosphere was set, defined by conflicting perceptions. Jon's mood was dominated by uncertainty as his father used the ornate but rusting knocker to announce their arrival.

As they were greeted, it became apparent that all was not well. Jon's aunt had a ghostly pallor, her eyes detached and glazed. Her frame was bent and obviously restricted in movement. As a result she was confined to a wheelchair and spoke with difficulty. Jon felt a certain sorrow.

In contrast with the exterior, the inside of the house was dingy and oppressive. The furnishings were sparse and appeared to belong to the distant past. There were coverings sprawled across the chairs and sofas, their patterns at odds with the surroundings. The walls were stained with nicotine, and the carpeting was frayed, worn by regular tread. The paintwork was splintered and chipped. Jon imagined that he was witnessing a scene from a period film as he surveyed the room before him. It was the antithesis of what he had expected. After the reassurance of the facade, it was very unsettling. They sat in the lounge where a series of abstract prints hung above the dilapidated fireplace. They were coated in dust, but the surreal landscapes were still visible. Their location broke the drabness, shooting into the dark. The abundance of ashtrays revealed numerous brands of extinguished weed, European and American.

At that moment a stocky, middle-aged man entered the room, a cigarette dangling from his mouth. Dishevelled and apparently preoccupied, his gait was unsteady, his actions cumbersome. Jon was instantly wary of this seemingly peculiar member of his family who introduced himself as David, in a voice slow and deliberate. The ash from his cigarette fell to the floor, but he seemed oblivious to it and began to light another from the stub. Jon began to view him with sympathy as he cut a pathetic figure, yet unnerving and mysterious. Jon was not sure as to whether David's enigmatic quality should be disturbed.

David turned on the television and sang a strange, atonal tune with real vigour, as the pictures flashed before him. There seemed to be some form of stimulus that he had keyed into. Quite what form it took was alien to his visitors. He then ran to the window and drew the curtains aggressively, as though commanded to do so. By complete contrast, he politely offered tea and explained that his beloved mother was suffering from cancer and her prognosis was poor. Jon's parents displayed no visible surprise and so Jon assumed that everyone had known of this situation bar him. He felt resentful but was rapidly distracted when David slammed the living room door, screeching as though a strangled bird. Jon's parents looked on in dismay whilst Jon felt tearful. He began to feel more saddened as time went by. This whole experience was testing, with little to gauge it by.

David's behaviour was unpredictable to say the least, as he wandered between the lounge and the kitchen. At times there was lucidity, but then confusion. There seemed to be no method, just random disturbance. Jon's aunt appeared sullen and withdrawn, a picture of suffering. The tea was served but had not been heated and Jon sat uncomfortably as his parents strove to make conversation. It was all rather hollow. The harder they tried to fill the gaps, the wider they became. David continued to alternate between an uneasy clarity and overwhelming melancholia. The whole scene evoked unhappiness and a feeling of desolation, which could not be escaped from. Jon desired some lightness and relief, wanting to return to the sanctuary of home, without the journey. It had all been rather overwhelming and he wanted it to end.

After what seemed an eternity, Jon's father indicated that it was time to depart. Jon felt relieved, but his concern for David was starting to make him agitated. He could not precisely locate the cause of this. He felt unsettled after David's peculiar behavioural display. As they moved into the hall to say their goodbyes, David beckoned Jon into the study. It became rapidly apparent that here much would be revealed, a special privilege for sure. Jon was to delve beneath the surface. As he entered the room of foreboding, Jon was staggered by an abundance of half-finished canvases, all revealing the subject of distress by way of life drawings and portraits. The assemblage was of the highest quality, the tonality of the sketches evocative, and the understanding of anatomy complete. There was evidence of manic energy, with inspiration taken from many artistic sources. Yet David's style was clear. This work needed to be hung proudly, not restricted by self doubt. It seemed like a doorway. Jon's feelings started to alter as he began to digest the content of what was before him. He acknowledged a transference of empathy for David displayed great courage in the face of adversity. David then opened a large, leather bound book which contained his poetry and verse, the beauty of which brought tears to Jon's eyes. It possessed a fragility and vulnerability that conveyed and explained so much about David's emotional makeup. It was poignant as it opened up his inner world. Jon was also struck by the beautifully presented italics, and interpretations of illuminated manuscripts. He felt privileged. A renaissance man for sure. So much was contained here, but at what cost? The currency appeared to be torment, but so much had become of it. At times David's words danced across the pages, and then stood still, in perfect contrast.

A soprano saxophone rested in the corner of the room, alongside various photographs of jazz legends. They were classic black and white shots, evoking the glory of Birdland in the early fifties. The smoke and the passion. The saxophone itself was gleaming, obviously a treasured possession. It symbolised a way of release, a tool of expression. David picked up the instrument, shaped a melody and made it sing. His tone was sweet, his delivery sparse. It was as though his thoughts were encapsulated in the sound. The acoustics of the room were slightly dead, but the emotion was not lost. Was this the music of the heavens, improvised by the gift of freedom? Jon hoped so, such was the impact. David then lowered himself carefully into a chair, clasping his head in silence.

After a while, David gestured to Jon to sit by him. Jon did so with a feeling of trepidation. David stared at Jon with vehemence, gripping his hand. He began to speak awkwardly, but he was rapidly becoming incoherent, and Jon had to focus intently, but to no avail.

Jon had witnessed David's images, heard his sound. The tone of the meeting was tinged with shades of blue and Jon could not escape this for he was powerless. Then just before the time of departure, David punched the side of his face and howled in pain.

Jon had to hold on, for in time he would become challenged by trials of the mind, just as David had been.

Yet when distilled, the meeting was full of woe for Jon had been warned by David, the man with scars that penetrated the deeper recesses.

So much to digest, the enormity of it all. A time

that warned of impending torment, delivered with uncanny precision. At the outset things had been grim and by the conclusion, much had been revealed. A great deal to absorb, and to decipher. Jon felt exposed, unearthing a focus, an inner drive. He respected David's words, their content, even whilst putting aside a stampede of emotions. Jon would travel to the cliff tops, in reflection, and toss the stone. And no one would ever see it land. Being with David that time was to remain with him forever.

The importance of that visit had transcended most other facets of Jon's life. He searched endlessly for sources of compassion. He yearned to laugh, be lost in pleasurable realms. This connected with a desire for simplicity where everything has its place. He knew the boundaries, and must not leave them. A web had been woven, to seize and ensnare. He needed to be away from the edge, where the current will not reach. Looking across to the flight of birds, Jon was now to face his isolation.

As the years passed Jon by, he had matured somewhat, probably more rapidly than most. Life had its routine and difficulties. At home he did not communicate with much relish, tending to keep himself to himself. Being an only child, in this household he was unused to the battles for supremacy that would be indicative of a larger family. He was often left to his own devices, and he had become self-sufficient, with no one to challenge his independence. At times his parents would howl with frustration, but to little effect. Jon wondered what it would be like to have an older brother, someone to look up to, perhaps share interests with. It was lonely sometimes. Who could he relate to? When there was no conversation at the meal table, or afterwards in the lounge, the greater the emptiness became. Emotion suppressed, feelings contained. This was the family.

When friends visited, they were met with enthusiasm, which would then fade. Jon found it a trial to maintain any momentum, in whatever area. There were developments but they were tinged with anguish. The invariable factors were that of distance, and he needed to discover a place where he was valued for his own particular eccentricities. Where idiosyncrasies were found a home. Such was Jon's desperate desire for acceptance.

Inside his bedroom there were many indications of seclusion, only the locks were not visible. Upon the exposed plaster were scribbles and scrawls, mainly indecipherable. Some took the form of patterns, highlighted by pen and wash. On the floor was a sea of literature, piled high. The bed's frame had been removed, leaving the mattress on the carpet. The tonality of the surroundings was rather bleak, and Jon would often huddle in the corner and listen to the voices. He had rearranged the furniture numerous times, never satisfied. He positioned bookcases and drawers in a manner that he believed would bring protection in case there was an onslaught for which he would now be prepared. The curtains could be drawn, light dimmed, only to display shadows cutting into the ensanguined, threadbare carpet. There were also slashes of ebony upon the haphazardly applied floor coverings.

Jon was an avid Lego construction fan, spending many hours designing and building; it was a source of great stimulation. Dotted around the room were completed works, alongside artefacts that pieced together chunks of memory. Included were an antique pair of binoculars that had provided Jon with a prop for war games. There were also sculptural items that he enjoyed to touch, caress. Within these darkened walls Jon found a certain solace.

Sometimes the hum of traffic from the nearby road would resemble a harmony and Jon would add his own rhythm. The poplar trees that lined the perimeter of the garden were visible from his window and Jon would watch them sway and tremble. They looked vulnerable, yet their roots were firm. The lawn had been invaded by moss, but when walked on, it felt like the softest of carpets. The borders had not been attended to for a long while and giant nettles pierced the air above. Jon focused on the tints of green, and appreciated what he saw.

Upstairs Jon held himself inside, within his haven, aware of and desiring space. He was attempting to divorce himself from the plateau, for little ever occurs there. He wanted to experience the extremes of existence. But one day he would yearn to enter an asylum, to escape the pain.

Although older, Jon was still in the playground. All around was activity. Contemporaries approached him but he pushed them away. He sat on the edge, observing. Everything seemed too busy, with too much to contemplate. There were swirls of dust, caught by the wind from time to time, like a scaled down desert storm. The bikesheds were occupied by kids keen for a drag, puffing frantically. Some girls were to be seen in the throws of furious argument, with no end in sight. The accumulation of movement and sound preoccupied Jon, with emotive arrows firing from every angle. An intensity was building, piece by piece, as an energy surge accompanied it. The boundaries of perception were converging, forming a focus like a razor's edge.

Jon considered himself to be planning something of great importance, even though he was unaware of its amplitude. But soon he would be. He felt he possessed a certain steadiness, much to his surprise, as he was normally a somewhat nervy individual. Was he now the great field marshal, plotting the attack? It would be directed towards himself however, but the preparation was just as exacting. The selection of protagonists was not to be hurried and the location was to be precise. Jon glanced at his watch, but time was in abundance. He felt as though he was floating above his own being, witnessing the formative steps of his own destruction. Before long, everything would be in place, with only the flare to commence action. Jon's vision was as transient as ever but he recognised its structure. As he scratched his forehead, he noticed beads of perspiration trickling down towards his eye brows. The moment was almost there.

Jon's body felt stiff and awkward as he rose to his feet. Approaching the middle of the playground, he made his way across the bleached grass. Jon counted to ten and strode forward into the centre of an improvised rugby pitch. There he deliberately knocked the largest and most unpredictable of the players to the ground. After the man mountain composed himself, he punched Jon full force in the face, the power of which splattered him in blood. Undeterred, Jon kicked wildly into the group surrounding him. This provoked a violent and hostile reaction. Jon was beaten to the floor, attacked from every angle. All he could see was a blur of fists and feet. He was covered by the shadow of the hostile mass. They appeared elongated, towering above. The assault was vicious, the flames roaring. Almost as a reflex he continued to thrust outwards, which only exacerbated the situation. He was sustaining blows all over, yet mentally he was in his own little capsule. The aggression appeared in slow motion, and he was viewing it all with detachment. The whole event had been manipulated, carefully and systematically. Despite this, he could not have braced himself completely against the reality. Eventually the offensive concluded. What would be the cost? Jon was left in a heap after being subjected to such brutality. He gazed at the blood-stained ground by his head and reeled in pain. He felt it right to the core. Slowly he moved his limbs and the reaction was the same. His clothing was torn, as was the inside of his mouth. With deliberation Jon attempted to sit up, but it was too much. Everyone had deserted him, the playground now barren. He really was on his own. His bruises were throbbing, the stage clear, where were they? Did no one care? Tentatively he opened his eyes wide, squinting at the soreness. It was all over now, he wanted to escape. Let the heavens pour, and they did. It was a relief, both soothing and as an anaesthetic. Jon let himself be drenched, losing any concept of time. He luxuriated in the feeling. When he became conscious, he dared to rise, and was able. He stretched out his arms and looked down on his bloodied body. But it did not matter. He was in the arena, the crowds dispersed.

A most intense feeling of joyousness flooded through his veins. He projected all his praise upwards and began to run, elevated and effervescent. Despite the incongruity of events, Jon had realised their purpose and now he had been blessed from head to foot. It had all been so necessary, but with so much to endure. Now it was over, time to revel, to soak in the relief. He bounced onto the pavement and hurtled off into the distance. He was exuberant, calling out as he ran. His clothes had turned to rags, his shoes split and crumpled. His tendons were taut, in anticipation. His direction was unclear and was unimportant. The energy delivered was plenteous as his stains were washed away. The path was laid out before him and he continued to follow it. His external condition was purified and the agony had ceased. He was lifted up, and advanced into the clouds.

The penance had been paid, but there was much to transcend and to confront. Courage was needed to live, to go beyond a life of conformity.

Jon sat on the edge of the hill, surrounded by bracken and insects in profusion. They cosseted him as did the seraphic. He had begun to travel, sucked in by the expanse. He was the voyager. Now let life begin.

LIVES WITHIN A LIFE

CHAPTER TWO – ART

By now Jon was in the last throes of the educative system. He felt weary, and frustrated. He was in no way prepared for, or receptive to, academia. His behaviour had become more and more erratic, and many of the tutors had no idea how to respond. The standard of his work was progressively slipping, despite his intellect. Somewhere there was a well of ability, but his lack of concentration and focus held him back. Jon did not belong to any social grouping and was seen by those in authority to drift in and out of contact with others. This was resented by some while others viewed him as an eccentric outcast, an object of ridicule and derision. He had taken to wearing torn, scruffy clothes, not to make any kind of statement but because they seemed appropriate. His hair was long and matted, his ears studded with fake gems. There were burn marks on his forearms, which no one dared enquire about. During break times he would race to the top of the playing field and roll cigar-sized cigarettes, smoking one after the other. His fingers were shades of burnt sienna. Jon often thought of David and his appetite for nicotine. Sometimes he was approached for a light, and he obliged, igniting his Zippo. But he would always return to himself. He would have been popular if only he had the confidence. In lesson time he was always dreaming, his thoughts wandering. His subjects had been chosen on his behalf by his parents. He had taken exception to this and it gave him more reason to drop out. Jon displayed a complexity that made him hard to understand.

The cloisters were a haven of calm and Jon would be seen there at times, deep in thought. Internally, he was preparing to open himself up in order to express his innermost emotions. Memories of days past were starting to emerge and he was taking heed. Jon was becoming aware of vivid images and violent colours that passed before his eyes. His imagination was to reveal structure, but within different confines. Everything Jon viewed was either a photograph, a painting, or a piece of sculpture. Regardless of medium, they captured the essence. From this foundation there would be many methods that expounded Jon's perception of nature, all highlighting the image. He found this exciting, a true stimulant. Jon took in the ranges of tonality, forms of architecture, the swaying of each tree, the effects of technology. He immersed himself in his surroundings and made that his point of study. All of these artistic elements combined to represent Jon's life. Quality of light was also to preoccupy, its variation influencing his own particular window of the world. To Jon, these were the essentials. And he would continue to explore, for this had reason. The transitory nature of the clouds drifted over, and he would watch them until they could hold no more. The pouring over brick work, patterns and routes, all improvised. Even the weaving of a web would lead the mind. What Jon required was somewhere to channel all of this dynamism, somewhere to learn. This was all so far from the tedium of his schooling. But maybe there was a way.

Up in the recesses of the art department was a

LIVES WITHIN A LIFE

teacher known for his unusual methods and approach. Normally when conversing with him, he did not appear to register. But then he would surprise those in his company with a pertinent retort. Jon had decided to go and speak to him with the hope of finding time to be guided in this field. So, at the end of the day he headed off to explain his situation.

After climbing several flights of stairs, Jon knocked on the art master's door. Typically, there was no reply. Jon hesitated and then repeated his attempt to gain entry to the office. Still nothing. Jon slowly opened the door to find the tutor lost in a recording of Wagner to which he was listening. He was understandably startled when he saw Jon standing before him. He turned his stereo off and apologised, which Jon regarded as unnecessary. The office was covered from wall to wall with Italian renaissance prints. A small cigar was smouldering in the ashtray. The whiff of stale smoke was not particularly pleasant, even to a smoker. Books by Hemmingway and Jung were visible on top of the worn surface of the desk. There were also black and white photographs of children, presumably his. The shelves were straining with the weight of volumes of reference. His hi-fi was in separate form, and obviously of some value. Apart from the Wagner on top of the pile, there were recordings of Billie Holiday and Muddy Waters. A clearly eclectic collection. Small animals fashioned in bronze surrounded the large notepad in the centre of the table. Spider plants hung perilously from the filing cabinets. Half burnt candles were dotted randomly. A certain fragility was displayed by the beautifully formed pottery. The glazes were sourced from metals, and shone when they caught the light. The room possessed an abundance of character, built up over the time it had been occupied. Jon was impressed.

The teacher turned round and asked Jon what he saw in a rainbow. Jon listed the colours, sensing that he needed to say more in response. He was right, for the tutor conveyed that it was more than a spectrum, it symbolised a radiance and was an example of natural phenomena. This was the crux of the questioning. To look beyond was something that Jon could relate to. Instinctively he started to explain his theories and notions in a rambling but revealing way. He felt safe and able to do so. Intuitively he knew that the man before him was an answer to much that was unresolved. He had listened to Jon intently and respected his opinions. Jon then asked if he might be given the opportunity to draw and paint in the department. He needed support, and hoped this tutor could provide it. Much to his relief the teacher agreed, although there would be no exam owing to the late stage the formal course had reached.

Jon was beside himself - what an opportunity he had been given! He wanted to learn, discover and realise. And now it would happen, he was sure. There was no time to waste. His first task was to put together a library, containing chronicles of history and style. Various artistic mediums were to be purchased and the mind's eye nurtured. He would need to study, with discipline. From this base, a tangible construction of Jon's visions could begin. He felt butterflies fluttering inside his stomach, such was his anticipation.

Today had been a tremendous boost, helping to sustain Jon's eagerness, his zest. He was concerned with more than the aesthetic and wanted to comprehend artistry as a whole. The complexities of mass and its relationship to its surroundings. Art was to broaden his view, such was the ever changing nature of existence. The clarity of line and form was displayed by the masters whose precision of draughtsmanship contained it completely. The anatomy of man and beast had been studied in order to understand the surface. Their architecture was all about space and balance. Proportion hewn from marble, with respect of the material. Jon was to appreciate and marvel at their vitality, their scope. They retained a humanity, from the primitive to the sophisticated. This was often communicated within a single pose.

All of this richness overwhelmed Jon but accelerated his passion for learning. It was a rapid journey, with many movements and styles left unexplored, but it gave him an adequate grounding to build on.

Jon's own perceptions paralleled the abstraction that prospered when he immersed himself in the geometric breakdown of objects. He was particularly interested in the idea of viewing something from several angles concurrently. The concept of recognising structures in space had taken him several steps further. This sense of space and volume was visible along intersecting planes and keyed into Jon's experiences of illusion and his juxtaposition of specific styles. To him it was all liberating, as were the variations on the theme. By showing several simultaneous motions, with elasticity and at times a certain violence, Jon had found a profusion of reference points.

The art of the dream world seemed to inform his waking state, creating its own visual language. Paranoid existence could be identified also, set against barren landscapes. Because the walls of the subconscious were being broken down, there was much to be revealed and so understood. And Jon was only at the beginning.

He was starting to appreciate that good draughtsmanship is the basis of inventive art. An inner eye to visualize, and the psyche utilised to acquire a knowledge of the science of drawing. On that determining principle, imagination and flair can be added. The balance of order and chance are also elements. To watch the forever changing quality of light over the mountain ranges, and then to transpose that onto canvas. The steely blues of the winter sky in contrast, revealing a magical tonality. Each mark etched in time, a visual diary to refer to. But as the years pass by, so skills improve, enabling the individual to convey their particular vision in entirety. Jon aimed to capture the whole, to become one with the skyscape. He spent hours at a time studying, losing himself in the expansive area of strongly figurative art. He was sometimes disturbed by any oppressive quality, because it reminded him of his own demons. But now he had found a method with which to try and cleanse his soul.

It was an opening to a new world, as Jon held the pastels, mixed the oils and set about creating his own representations. At this point he had never forgotten David. Those life studies' forlorn nature, and their aching quality. All lost in that insular existence, never to be properly appreciated outside of it. His mind was constantly assimilating whilst his imagination pushed him onwards to fresh and challenging boundaries. Jon was preoccupied with the thrust of manic energy, and its power. He wanted to visit different lands, see a thousand faces, cross the deepest oceans.

Before Jon was a blank piece of paper, a vantage point from which he was to convey his own experiences. He was concerned with recording relevant images, and he chose to do so by viewing reality from the edge. He aspired towards those who possessed the most vitality, thinking inventively, taking risks. His desire was to be an expressive innovator, one who pushed to extremes but retained the judgement to withdraw just before total immersion. Jon wanted to fly in the clouds, take in the expanse of blue, break through the beams of light. He was to be the starchild, taking in the stratospheric and ethereal. To be able to retain that resolve, to hold onto a certain belief that one day he would reign victorious.

The first project involved perspective, vanishing points and associated theories. Jon had to align the fading brick work and window frames from his view point. It required concentration to which he applied himself. The light was scorching, revealing every grain. The next time it was to be interiors, still lives, the arrangement of objects. Jon was learning the use of textural oil, the wash of water colours, the blending of pastel and chalk, and darker tones filled with ink. In life classes he followed the curves of the body, the sinews and muscle groupings, every angle a different picture. He was becoming aware of the fine, obsessive art of illustration and the discipline and professionalism of graphic design. Jon enjoyed the manipulation of all mediums and was particularly at home with ceramics, at the wheel, or sculpture.

It was as though a whole new sense of purpose had been awakened in him. It brought with it a feeling of invigoration, as patterns and arrangements took on new meaning, the tiniest of nuances building up an intricate kaleidoscope.

Jon's sketch pad was always by his side, to record a visual diary. He would soon amass many of these, full of ideas, starting points and influences. The momentum had to be maintained, the mind open and predisposed towards artistic endeavour. Many of Jon's contemporaries were sports devotees, but his passion lay in the arts. This left him open to mockery, but it was of no concern. For his reason to progress was established.

Jon looked down onto the shore, to the boulders that braved the elements and he caught that moment, his hand guided. For now he could see it

LIVES WITHIN A LIFE

all.

It had started quite by accident. Jon was out walking, taking in the air. He was striding with vigour, his head moving to the beat that existed within him. The obligatory sketch book was in his hand, held together by an elastic band. It was a pleasant day and before long Jon decided to sit on a dry stone wall by the parkland, and to enjoy the warmth. He surveyed the surrounding area, from the roadside to the tree tops. Nearby was a small row of cottages that had been converted from an old riding stables. They were very attractive, particularly their sandy stonework and immaculate gardens, laid out with flowers in orderly rows, displaying riots of colour. The windows were full of exotic plants, forming their own enclosure around the glass.

As Jon continued to observe, a skylight was opened in the loft of the house nearest to him. Jon had always dreamed of setting up a studio in an attic, where he could work undisturbed. It would have stripped pine floorboards, white-washed walls and plenty of space. As Jon contemplated the idea, the most wondrous sound began to emanate from the window opening. It sent a chill down his spine. It was the strain of a trumpet, set to a lush orchestration, with echoes of flamenco harmony and a sparseness that were to dazzle and bewitch. Jon held up his head, his eyes misty. The harmonies were carried by the rhythm and resonance of the bass. They twined, and then reverberated. The varying tempo always caught the swing. This was musical greatness, although Jon could not identify it. He immersed himself in the sunlight and the sweetest of sounds.

Unbeknown to him, a man had stepped out onto the front lawn and glanced at Jon inquisitively. But Jon was totally enraptured in the music, to him it was the most complete source of inspiration. He was awoken from his trance with a start when the man approached him, asking his business. All Jon could find to say was the truth, he was listening to the overspill. The man then explained that it was his recordings that were the cause of his fascination. Jon was full of eagerness again and wanted to know all about the sounds. With that question still unanswered, he was ushered into the house and up a spiral staircase. As he entered the top room, he immediately noticed a huge pair of speakers in the far corners. There was an armchair between them, and shelves full of music. As Jon turned to face the owner of the house, in his mind's eye all he could see was David.

Jon then apologised for any apparent hesitancy and began to explain how he had felt when he heard this colossal work. It was exactly as the gentleman had experienced at around Jon's age, and it too had made a huge impression. There was so much to talk of, to enquire about. There was more to this supposedly chance meeting than was immediately obvious. The man was as surprised as Jon that this situation had occurred at all, but since it had, it was time to capitalise. They sat down with iced tea and sandwiches and spoke of be-bop, The Birth of Cool, Mahler, modal progressions, Debussy, electric Jazz, Fusion, Wagner. It all went deep into the night, with disc after disc hitting the turntable. A door of enlightenment was opening, and Jon was hurtling through. He was witnessing the spontaneity of rhythmic figures, impressions, and collages of sound that equated with his own internal compositions. He listened to music where convention was blown apart. Phrases encompassing a multitude of emotions all condensed into sweet concord, like musical alchemy. It transcended spheres of courage, or enquiry. As the sounds filled Jon's ears, words formed within his inner psyche, for these passages were to shape a fusion that would go beyond the lucid qualities of that day. More than he could know.

For now Jon was no longer satisfied, as his desire was overpowering to the extent that he did not want just to hear these sounds, he wanted to make, create and shape them. He recalled David's soprano saxophone, lying in the corner, as he looked at his new friend. They both recognised a collective yearning to reach out to those cathedrals of sound, for that is what they had become. They could reach pinnacles with which to pierce the skin of emotional extremes.

Although Jon was becoming aware of an increasing sense of purpose, there was much to study in preparation. Maybe it would take a lifetime? He sat at the keyboard in order to discover the chords that were swelling within, one by one. The repetition wore him down, but he did not relent. The structures and language of musicality had to be unearthed. At times only a cacophony could be heard inside, and sometimes the wealth of notes was intimidating, but he persisted. As Jon continued, he learnt more about the role of punctuation, in building a sense of drama. He could hear the soaring intensity of a full orchestra. He learned also to curb his natural impatience, for the process had to be taken stage by stage. He found his dexterity was improving as he produced flurries of notes and practised scales. He allotted time each day, and adhered to this rigidly. At times of rest he would listen to new recordings, provided by the man at the cottage who was following Jon's progress with interest. Jon's parents were pleased also, because of the effect these creations were having on their lost son. They would pop into the music room from time to time, and smile, reassured. Mealtimes had a new air of lightness, even frivolity. They hoped life would become more stable and less trying, for they really did love Jon, but did not know how to approach him. Maybe now the tide was turning. For this they had earnestly prayed, often in the depths of despair.

His father had likened watching the deterioration of his son's mental state to being a powerless bystander as Jon stood facing the traffic on the wrong side of a streaming motorway. He had felt inadequate, as did Jon's mother. She was the dominant one of the two and had at times lost her temper, which in retrospect, she wished she had not. But to witness an only child become so unapproachable and alienated was too much to bear. They provided what they could materially but this, of course, could never be enough. They had always retained high hopes for Jon academically, but these had been dashed. Seeing him so alone, and so visibly agitated, the two just wanted to hold him and remove all the misery. Jon's father was prone to depression and this was exacerbated by his concern for his son. He felt responsible. His distance, remoteness, was often born out of an inability to deal with his own feelings. Jon's mother wanted to approach the situation in a practical manner, but this often stepped beyond realms that were attainable. Matters were evolving into something more ingrained and complex. The household often felt cold and unaccommodating, with three individuals out of step with each other. Would it take an extreme incident to bring them together? Perhaps a more collective effort was required.

Now the house was full of music as Jon became more adept at his chosen craft. His father could sometimes be heard whistling in the background, with a broad smile spread across his ageing face. But despite this, he could not remove his fear for Jon's future. What would become of him? Would there ever be any consistency to counter his ingrained patterns of behaviour? He needed an answer. He yearned for this. For Jon was his flesh and blood.

Back to the piano, where Jon had remained seemingly for an eternity, ever formulating his sound. The keys were now familiar, the theories tangible. With this the peaks would be attainable, and there would be an assembly of emotional significance and intimacy: the synthesis of exploration and location. He could see it all in shapes, the internal imagery cutting to the quick. Curiously, Jon could not read a note, it was all contained in his head. He would write the sweetest lullaby and, in turn, the most explosive symphony, with the roll of kettle drums on the horizon. Jon needed to fill voids with dynamism, to relate to the strings and choirs that raged in his head. He could conduct with passion, project an exuberance that was sourced from his inability to connect with the simply ordinary. For from his vantage point Jon could see the definition of the truly extraordinary. He had been blessed with the gift to capture a certain vulnerability that exists in all of us. He wanted to incorporate humour, pain, elevation and anguish, and transpose it all. To aim high was the only way. The question in the back of Jon's mind was where to place the impending emotive surge. Would it be from the rooftops, or upon the mountain side over the valleys? Would he need thousands of watts or would it be subliminal? For now he left those questions unanswered.

Jon was aware, however, that he needed to become proficient on another instrument. He loved to feel the pulse of the bass, and when it resonated, rippling through the forests. It pushed the beat forwards and solidified the rhythm. You had to lock into the groove and become immersed in the syncopation. The upright bass has been in existence for more than 300 years, and now Jon was going to indulge in its heritage. He wanted to vary the dynamics, by bow, picking and finger style. The freedom of a fretless fingerboard also appealed. He wanted a meaty tone and the room to interplay with other instruments. Jon was to break down the harmonies, and to utilise them to create a wall of sound. He was also aware of the importance of harmonic intonation, to possess the necessary precision. Brilliance comes through mistakes, a time to discover, and Jon endeavoured to stretch beyond any constraints of convention. For as Jon walked along meandering paths, he was followed by his shadow. But he chose to confine that darkness to the challenge of acoustic energy.

The bedroom walls were lined in ebony with pillar box red piping. They were now bare apart from an early photograph of David. He was standing on a village green, resplendent in his cricket whites. Jon would often lie on his bed and stare at it and think of his words. For in his mind they had been carved in granite.

In the corner of Jon's room stood his three-quarter size double bass, a little worn, yet still full of presence and character. He referred to it as the mammoth, because of its huge sound. His finger tips were hardened from playing it, as he had exercised across the strings. He would hammer and pop, slide and modulate, varying pitch and volume. Jon's aim was to become as one with the fingerboard, a wholly natural extension, for he was truly motivated and driven. His voice would now be carried by the clouds, conveying an accumulation of both wired intensity and vulnerable tenderness. The formation of chords, the shapes of the hand, the attack and accent. There were times when Jon would weep at the profundity. Piece by piece the instruments interlocked, building a wider, panoramic picture. Their interaction was helping to define Jon's dream.

He would often contemplate the amalgamation of sound and vision with literature, to tell his story. But he needed to be believed in, for someone to give him support. He was essentially a loner, drifting on the edge of society, learning to live with rejection. At times he would even consider a life on the streets, so avoiding all contact.

But now Jon was composing, and prolific in his quest. He had to bring all of this creative vigour into a reachable outlet as it would be of no use if it were not attainable to others. Jon felt as though he was ascending to an uplifted state. From that pinnacle he would reveal the arena in which to perform his work; where all sensations would connect and flow from one body to the next.

Despite his creative immersion, Jon was still a troubled soul. Outside of his musical realms he would listen to voices, and they would interfere and penetrate with venom. Sometimes they would take the form of indescribable noise, but mainly a commanding voice could be heard, as two others talked about him as though they were in a padded cell, bringing endless mocking and snide laughter. At times there were whole dramatic passages enacted, with a multitude of foreign tongues. They would emanate initially from the core of his brain and then expand, becoming more and more intrusive. Their relentlessness wore Jon down until he was broken. He would walk along road and path, and they were forever inside of him, slowly grinding away.

He would also experience satanic projections, with disfigured faces erupting from the paving stones. Glistening bars would appear, trapping him in time. Bodies decomposed in front of his petrified eyes. He could see beneath the skin tissues to the rotting bone. Insects would crawl all over his skin as he howled in agony. Walls and ceilings closed inwards, crushing without mercy. Jon would witness his own body, and watch it being mutilated, torn apart. Inanimate objects would come alive, taking absolute control, issuing orders and demands. Jon would be held captive for hours, days even. Distorted visions of familiar persons would also appear, as grotesque deviants. Jon's arms were covered in scars and burns where he had been commanded to cut himself up, severing the arteries. He had flung himself into the path of speeding cars, intent on self-destruction. This was the way that he was led. The seeds had been sown the day he left the playground all those years ago. Those initial murmurings had built in intensity, taking more and more of a hold. He was becoming a helpless victim.

Now the fragmentation had set in, shattering Jon's consciousness, leaving him to live a waking nightmare. Tables and objects were to be seen gyrating and breathing with their own set of lungs, of independent volition. Sometimes they would prance wildly around, like some bizarre piece of animation. Jon had made friends with the bricks in the walls, they were strong, steady, and could be held onto. In contrast to the bricks were the birds, signifying his freedom. He would watch them from the window in full flight and dream. He would long for them to take him away. He had even built a shrine for his friends, made from stone and feathers, held together by the moist soil from the earth. There were pieces of fruit laid around it, symbolising his downfall, just as mankind had itself succumbed to temptation.

Jon's resolution was to remain intact, however. He was aware that his soul had been contaminated at the point of conception. Because of the creative fusion that would bring collective compassion to those suffering, he was under relentless attack. This was about his potential; he had been placed on this earth to fulfil a particular role. Such was its enormity, the demons were placed by the devil in order to destroy the source that was to be the catalyst and generate positive energy. Yet he would continue to construct the relevant pieces, these being elements of imagery, literature and music. They would form a bond that would transcend all. Those abstracted and forlorn would be brought together and healed. Only Jon and the Lord were aware of the reach of this deliverance. Jon would often call for the voices to leave him, the visions to dissipate. He dreamt of climbing to the top of the dome of release, to look down, and the world would be complete. The orchestra would roar in agreement, with the illumination filling the sky. Despite all the difficulties he would remain on the right path, focusing on the truth.

He had spent so many hours in conversation, interacting with the commentaries in his head, which no one else could hear. But to Jon it was not an alien experience, it encompassed his life. He longed for a cessation of the trials of the mind and be taken to a place where he could lie with only the light before him. That was all. For he was the walking wounded.

Then, quite unexpectedly, Jon was taken to a land of opportunity where all the pieces would fall into place. The timing could not have been better.

He had taken to visiting the local music shop to check out the latest instruments and related technology. He had become a familiar face there and the owners let him spend time playing the keyboards and guitars. He was a good advertisement for their wares. Other local musicians would pop in and they would chat about the latest sounds over coffee and cigarettes. It was an exciting time. It was during one of those sessions that Jon was approached by a saxophonist who had been on the road for several years. Jon used to experiment with different bass guitars and upright basses and this man liked his sound. He asked if Jon had any commitments, which provoked a certain intrigue. Jon responded by explaining that he had lots of time on his hands, that he was waiting for something to develop, and that now it seemed something would.

Jon was asked to fill a gap in a band that were to be residents in a club in Amsterdam. The money was adequate and accommodation was provided. The music was a mixture of blues and mainstream jazz, with a bit of added wildness at times, and room for improvisation. The venue held about 200 people on a good night and the group were to play five nights a week. The days were free of commitment, so providing time to familiarise oneself with the city. Jon had all the necessary equipment at home, which could be transported, so all he needed to do was pack his bags. The fact that someone believed in him meant so much and as a consequence Jon could feel himself rushing up to a high. To be able to travel and play was good news, so he confirmed that he wanted the gig and rushed home.

Jon's parents did not want him to leave as they were most concerned for his welfare. It seemed so unstable an existence, and far away. But as they absorbed their son's enthusiasm, they realised they had to let him go. It was a chance and they had to let him take it. They so much wanted him to be happy, and they recognised his gift, but there would be many tears when he departed.

And so Jon left. At the airport his mother and father held him close as his flight was called. Jon then walked into the tunnel and was gone. As the plane ascended Jon looked out through the window, and although his parents were out of sight, he continued to wave, thinking of their love.

Up in the air Jon watched the candy floss skies, the brilliance of the sunlight. For him, it was the dawning of a new age. He intended to take in the cosmopolitan flavour of Amsterdam, with its galleries, theatre land and architecture; it was all there waiting for him.

Jon had been given an address where he would be introduced to the rest of the band. As he threaded his way through a myriad of backstreets, he heard a profusion of lively conversation, whilst witnessing individuals wearing a broad spectrum of vibrantly coloured clothes. On first impressions Jon liked the feel of this place.

Before long he saw the saxophonist approaching, a Gitanes dangling from his mouth. Jon waved and walked towards him. They were pleased to see each other. After dispensing with the trivia of small talk, they took a taxi to a small hotel, located off the beaten track. The rest of the band were hanging out at the bar and Jon was introduced to them. There was a drummer, keyboard player, guitarist, the saxophonist already familiar, and the engineer. They were all considerably older than Jon, looking pretty worn and haggard, the price to be paid for all that time on the road no doubt. A fresh round of beers arrived, foaming over. Jon was unsure what to say, since talking in a group had never been easy. The saxophonist passed the source of his blue smoke around, whilst Jon tucked into his halfzware tobacco. All the equipment was to arrive soon and they were then to spend a few days rehearsing the set list.

After a few drinks conversation relaxed. They spoke of their influences, the way they would approach the music. They were all on the same wavelength, and they wanted to capture the atmosphere in a way that had meaning for them all, to convey that elusive lyrical quality.

By now the excitement was building up and Jon was itching to get into the rehearsal room. He wanted to prepare and reach new musical horizons, to be part of a sonic synthesis where in his head were beautiful layers, waiting to be placed into the overall scene: a reflection of the times, the taste of the city, the heaving metropolis. There was a vibration to be captured, a pulse running through the veins. Jon's fellow musicians were to become more than companions off the stage, and would take him into an interactive nucleus when performing. There would be no need for words and Jon clung on in anticipation.

He had to try to control the noise inside, in order to combat the internal cacophony that would tear him into tiny pieces. He needed to be able to sculpt pillars of sound that could transcend all. Often he would rub his hands all over his head, straining for the convergence of energy with which to overcome the pain of savage, persecutory screams. However, after several days and nights of persistence, the tightness and interaction with the other players was within his grasp. The chords tore into the soul, as did the double bass drum beat, a riff on the stratocaster and the wail of the horn. It prompted a cohesion as various arrangements were explored and worked upon. The interplay was telepathic and Jon had impressed them with his skill. In turn he used the music to distract himself from the warfare that raged in his head. He was capitalising as intended and now he would take in all the excitement, for his place was established.

The first night was fraught with apprehension. This was the longed for opportunity to communicate with an emotional clarity that the collective believed they could attain. But the players were to be seen pacing, visiting the toilets with alarming frequency and chainsmoking. Their hands were trembling in agreement, creating animated silhouettes against a vivid backdrop. The tension was clearly palpable. Before long, the venue started to fill and there was a crescendo of chatter and voices. The bar area was full of sweaty bodies ordering their drinks in anticipation of the imminent concert..

It was now eight thirty and the group knew the time had come to make their entrance. They had to negotiate the short distance from the corridor that connected the dressing room to the stage. The saxophonist led them to their positions, and played a short scale. There were four strikes of the high hat and the night began. They possessed a big sound and it went down well. There was the appropriate rhythmic punctuation, the romance of the play between the saxophone and the fretless bass' fingerboard. The lead guitar created textural layers that began to soar as the guitarist's fingers raced up and down the instrument's neck. There were cheers of appreciation, including some for the self-penned tunes, much to the group's delight. The audience's feet were tapping, their hands clapping; the atmosphere was electric. This was the real high, embracing the band whilst connecting with their artistic sensibilities. They were all pouring with sweat, their concentration intense. Jon would sway with his bass, stamping out the rhythm. He was pushing forth to new boundaries, his eyes closed, relying on an intrinsic feel, which was evident and in abundance. At times he almost forgot about the audience, such was the depth of his focus. But when he did see them surrounding his skinny frame, he could not help smiling. He was able to sustain the energy levels for which he was thankful. The performance was draining, but in a wonderfully satisfying way.

When the night drew to a close and the crowd had dispersed, the band were all still singing and they exchanged hugs, somewhat overwhelmed by their exploration. They were shining like the stars above.

By now Jon was used to the routine that his life dictated, and on the whole he was content. He was able to indulge in the extremes of virtuosity as the projection of his own sound was well defined.

LIVES WITHIN A LIFE

But there was danger on the horizon, in the form of substances that seemed attractive but would ultimately cause mental derangement. Life on the road provoked the need to sustain the highs of performance and all around were freely available chemicals, but to indulge in their distorted reality would cause Jon to lose his sense of reason.

Despite this, Jon retained the inspiration to paint and construct. His room at the hotel was too small and impractical for his intentions but there was an empty attic nearby that would be perfect. He felt a need to create during the day as well as the evening. With a little negotiation the loft was his, he only had to pay a nominal amount for its use. He stretched numerous canvases and commenced his visual journey. The light was good and he could work undisturbed. There would be much abstraction as he followed his visionary expedition, such was the nature of his wandering perceptions.

Jon would mix the pigment with his fingertips, build up its consistency and try and translate the images that terrorized him in both his waking and sleeping hours. These hallucinations would leap out of the walls and fragment, and Jon would sit, huddled in the corner watching, begging for the brutal torture to cease. At night he played, as though on automatic pilot, so providing consistency in a creative sense. But a haze would always ensue, and it scared him. Jon was drained, but still wanting to invent.

His boards and fabric were covered by intense washes, textures created by oils, mixed with sand and pebbles and huge splashes of gloss. Ungainly lumps of cannabis were by his brushes and their consumption would sometimes induce colossal visions. There was a vulnerability in Jon's inner mind which was exploited by the drug. Most of the people around him smoked resin and he had succumbed. Initially it had helped him to open up and relax. After performing, it had become a necessity, but soon Jon was becoming lost in his own dreams, or predominately, nightmares. Sometimes he would smoke and paint until the next morning, and felt as though he could fly from the loft hatch. He would follow the thermal trails of aircraft and they would dance across his field of vision, and at times he would converse with the enemy, the devil within. He had begun to think that the drugs would take the edge off, ease the pain. He wanted to see the expanse before him and to capture this with every mark or stroke. At times he would walk the streets for hours, oblivious to risk. He was responding to commands that sent him on crazed trajectories. Jon would rest by the lamp posts, clamber through fencing, lost in his own little adventures. The music from the evenings would resonate in his head, but he was losing touch with reality. He was travelling into the distance and becoming fooled by the drug, a slave to it. It was rapidly transforming into an addiction, resulting in Jon forming an insidious dependency.

The band members thought Jon's behaviour was becoming increasingly irrational and disturbed. His conversations appeared unhinged and bizarre in their content. He was unkempt and prone to rambling, without any sense of what was outside his own internal world. He caused deep concern in his fellow players who now really cared about him, but also saw him as a liability. They could not afford any mistakes professionally and Jon was becoming more and more unreliable. His technique was still of a high standard, but his sense of placement was diminishing. The others decided to keep a close check on him, in the hope that he could hold himself together.

Jon's meanderings were becoming more extreme and he could not see where they were leading. He was out on a limb, racing ahead towards self-destruction as his foundations were weakening by the day. There were huge beats in his head of which he could not escape, and as a consequence he had secretly started to mutilate himself. When he had first indulged in this behaviour, he enjoyed the pain, but ultimately he thought he deserved it. The concept of penance was returning for Jon remembered the blood on the playground floor. To escape he would visualise surfing over the rooftops as though he was a bird. By now his studio was bursting with canvases, all revealing facets of his identity, the shattered pieces of a lost self. They were lined up in chronological order, displaying a diary of images representing the defined periods of his life. There were dreamscapes, bleeding skies, stretched tendons, expressions of anguish, all captured by strokes and marks, some deliberate, others more subliminal. Jon would soar into the early hours, at times when the lunar cycles could influence mood, leaving him to bark at the moon. Sporadic periods of silence would be broken by the scurrying patter of diseased rodents, barely contained by the inadequate drainage systems beneath. The weaving of the fabric, carrying the weight of oil and pigment, would only go to convey the tensions and cataclysmic pressures of Jon's sad, tortured existence. But his savage imagery would tear into the heart and soul and Jon was only just holding on. He felt that his work could be taken before some improvised altar, only for himself to be taken and sacrificed. He travelled through hidden doorways, entering weird, challenging but provocative realities, only occasionally to return to relative normality. Jon desired to leave something permanent, something that could withstand the force of demonic attack. When all the elements were fused together to create patterns that would not be lost as the seasons changed. Jon wanted to rise to the peak, stretch out his arms and embrace the world without fear or regret. He needed to fall into the supportive waves of the ocean's blue expanse, in order to progress devoid of mark and scar.

At times Jon would sleep in his studio until the afternoon, exhausted by his frenetic activity. He needed to find a place in which to rejuvenate and revitalise. His parent's letters were left by the door, unopened. Blocks of wood were strewn across the floor and had been arranged into a kind of fortress with which to protect his dwindling spirit. His state of mind was splintering and speeding downhill, with nothing to stop it. It would not be long before all he could hear was a cacophony, which signalled the onset of something dark and threatening. The detonation in his head overrode the pulse of the city, and it seemed relentless.

LIVES WITHIN A LIFE

Jon spent many hours located in the pavement cafes, filling his little black book with observations conveyed by verse and prose. These were accompanied by pencil studies captured when his eye was objective enough to see with clarity. But as Jon wandered into a labyrinth of alleyways, he was being sucked into a vortex where persecution reigned, and he was left, screaming in submission.

Not even the birds could reach him now, he was too far gone. Jon was plunging into the abyss, a place where the mind would be contorted beyond recognition, where nothing could be understood.

Jon stood up at the window ledge and called out to the city, hollering and crying. But there was no sanctuary to be found.

The saxophonist burst into the attic room and hurtled across its slippery floor, almost losing his footing, such was his sense of urgency. Jon had not shown up to the gig, and he had sensed that something was wrong. His worst fears were realised as he found Jon sprawled out over a blanket, covered in blood. He had written expletives on the wall after severing his arteries, and was now unconscious, his wounds gaping. An ambulance was called, and Jon's wrists and neck were bound with an improvised dressing. His skin was of a deathly pallor, and the saxophonist was shouting and screaming in an attempt to keep him alive. He cradled Jon's head in his arms, stroking his hair. He had to live, he had to! Jon just lay there, his eyes motionless, his body immobile.

Outside, a siren could be heard, and the paramedics raced up the stairs beginning immediate treatment. Jon was placed on a stretcher and taken to hospital. The saxophonist was frantic, blaming himself for not sensing the depths of Jon's despair. As the ambulance careered up the street he prayed for Jon's survival. To let him live, to breathe. But no one was to blame, for nothing could have prevented Jon's actions, such was his state of mind. He had deteriorated to such an extent that nobody could see how far he had fallen. Now it was up to the doctors to bring him back.

In the corner of the loft was Jon's beloved double bass, and after the commotion had eased the saxophonist walked over to it, running his hands over the wood. He plucked a string and reminded himself of Jon when times were good, when he had caught Jon's eye from across the stage, and saw it sparkle. The angels were dancing over his pupils, his laughter lines etched although in stone. Those bony fingers had created their own magic. He had so much talent, so much to give. To think that it could all end now was too much to contend with, the loss would be too great. He broke down and wept.

Jon awoke several days later, hooked up to all manner of machines. He cut a pathetic figure, dwarfed by the technology surrounding him. All he could recall was a ball of redness, which had enveloped him.

LIVES WITHIN A LIFE

And then darkness, such terrible darkness. A bombardment of deepest ebony, from which there was no escape. He was weak, finding it increasingly difficult to breathe. There were several nurses by his side and they were very attentive. However, Jon wanted to know what had happened to him and then, as he surveyed the immediate vicinity, he caught sight of his arms. They were wrapped in dressings, and he felt the stitches pull as he moved. At this point he became distraught, demanding answers. What had occurred beneath those fateful clouds? Before long a doctor arrived, and he bent down, holding Jon's hand. With a certain detachment he explained everything.

Jon realised how close he had come to death, and was left feeling brutalised and confused. Part of him still desired an end to it all but this co-existed with a sense of relief. Would he really have gone? And where would he have gone to? He was to spend more time on the ward, with plenty of time to consider these questions. But for now they could not be answered.

Jon awoke one morning after a fitful night, his bed wringing wet. He had experienced an episode of the nocturnal terrors that had afflicted him more and more frequently since his suicide attempt. It was then that a realisation suddenly hit him. He had not adhered to any Biblical teachings for what seemed an eternity. He had not even thought of it as he had been so far away from any sense of positive spirituality. Jon considered the possibility that this fresh awareness was a sign, for it seemed that he had been travelling endlessly without guidance. He felt that he had plunged towards the pits of hell. It was then that he sat up and called up to the heavens, and prayed in earnest. He needed to be forgiven, to be understood. It was at that point that two orderlies entered his room and Jon sensed an air of foreboding. With no element of choice, they were to take him away, kicking and screaming.

Jon was to be detained but what was his wrongdoing? He had endured a life of suffering and as a consequence Jon was to withdraw, entering a bizarre, tortured world. He had come so close to death but was saved from self-destruction. Now he needed to reaffirm his role on this planet, to think of the creative elements that would reshape his identity.

Maybe there would be another way, using different methods, an alternative vision. But now he had to learn how to survive. His liberty was to be taken away, and the cell doors locked. If only he could be heard, for someone to tend his aching wounds, to bring an end to the spiral downwards. Jon called out in despair as the rapidly darkening sky encompassed him.

LIVES WITHIN A LIFE

CHAPTER THREE - LIFE

Jon had been flown back to England at his parent's request. They were beside themselves when they heard the news and wanted to be with him and share the burden of his heavy heart. However, they could not help thinking that it had all been inevitable. They too felt his descent but they would not leave him, such was their resolve. Their love for Jon was abundant but they had to take him to the asylum, their choice removed. This tore into their very flesh, to stand by whilst he was committed.

Jon had been put on a secure unit and was held there by law, restricted by the Mental Health Section powers. He was stripped of his dignity, and was watched like a hawk. There was no privacy and he felt that the orderlies could read all the messages that his mind projected. He was given copious quantities of medicine, which left him under heavy sedation. Jon felt that his limbs were weighed down by concrete. The effort required to move seemed colossal. He found it difficult to gesticulate, with little control over his muscles. His psychomotor functions were severely affected and, as a consequence, he would frequently shake violently, his tongue expanding and saliva dripping onto the floor. He also had difficulty speaking, as his lips trembled and quivered, and he would tread with his feet like a cat on wool. He felt like a freak in a Victorian side show. Jon could hear the humiliating insults coming from all directions. He would stagger and sway, as though intoxicated. He was at times incontinent and felt ashamed and desperate. He could not sink any further for he was in the depths.

The drugs came in the form of injections and tablets and when Jon resisted them being administered, heavy nurses would appear out of nowhere and bring him to the ground. He would feel the jab as the needle punctured the skin. Jon would try to escape the medicinal torture as he felt a victim, rather than a patient. The regime was unrelenting and he wanted to escape from it all. He was the prisoner, languishing in a stripped-down cell.

The tables and chairs on the ward were bolted to the floor, the cutlery dispensed and then counted after every meal. The television was behind reinforced plastic which also covered the windows and the observation area. The staff would remain behind this for hour after hour, with contact minimised. But when there was any threat of violence, they would suddenly appear, forming a wall around the aggressor. He or she would then be man-handled into time-out, a cell empty apart from a bare mattress on the floor. There were no windows, and no light. When Jon found himself in there, it seemed the darkest place on earth. The outbursts that provoked this form of detention were motivated by frustration, the injustice of it all. But Jon was unable to find any solace, which only exacerbated his sense of isolation. There seemed to be such a degree of mistrust displayed by the staff towards those who were incarcerated; those who had been taken away, who could not run into the fields of corn that Jon recalled from his early years.

LIVES WITHIN A LIFE

There were no locks on the toilet doors, and patients would intrude as it was being used, such was the lack of privacy. At bath times, two people would bathe along side each other, with a nurse watching their every move. There were eyes everywhere and it was hard to imagine the cumulative effect of all this on Jon's mind, such was the level of indignity. He longed for simple things, such as walking in the park, or cycling along the country lanes. He reflected on times in Amsterdam when he was on the stage, immersing himself in the orchestral transposition. He could communicate through the bending of a string, or the crescendo of a soaring blues scale. But this period was all so far away now, almost as if it had occurred in a different lifetime. A time of lost dreams, now alien and distant.

Sometimes Jon would curl up in a corner, not wanting to see or hear anyone. When approached, he would only become more entwined by the inner workings of his mind. He was still in a precarious position, not far from descending over the edge. He was overwhelmed by vulnerability only to witness the laceration of his skin as he roared with pain. Jon saw beetles crawling all over his eyes, scorpions in his hair and serpents ready to devour his naked flesh. He was captive.

The nurses were a mixed bunch, some caring, others lazy and uninterested. The latter were in the majority. There was also the heavy mob, only a phone call away. They were there to do the restraining, and at times to indulge in their sick passion for inflicting a few bruises. Jon despised them and used to joke at times that when the revolution came, they would be the first to go. They would be made to pay for their cruel aggression and unrelenting sadism.

The psychiatrist assigned to Jon's case lived in another world. He had no empathy or practical advice to give. To him Jon was just a case number and he showed no interest in Jon's story, only a gaping void when it came to responding to his emotive alarm. Jon was left to contend with his loneliness whilst yearning for someone to rescue his soul from the harshness of life.

Most of the conversations aired during the weekly patient appraisals were centred on medication, with no room to discuss feelings. The psychiatrist did not know Jon at all yet he held the key to his freedom. On the occasions when Jon would shout in frustration, he was carted off into seclusion to cool down. He would lie there counting the hours, such was the unrelenting gloom that encompassed. Jon learnt to rely on his instinct, just to survive. But the bars of confinement were always visible.

Jon did not want any visitors for the first few months, including his mother and father. This had caused them distress but Jon could not cope with the intimacy of family togetherness. He felt that it would be easier if no one saw him. But as time went on, his feelings changed and he began to long for some outside contact.

When his parents arrived for the first time, the atmosphere was tense as Jon considered himself to be languishing in a jail, with all hope of liberty stripped from him. He was still being surveyed intently by the staff, their eyes burning his flesh. They all found it difficult to communicate and Jon's mother was reduced to tears. She attempted to take his hand, but he pulled it away. He was not ready for physical contact, for all he knew was the repression instigated by the orderlies. They would take him into the dungeons, kicking and screaming. But Jon did not know the nature of his crime. He was a victim of the system.

Jon's father's features were creased as he looked around the ward, obviously troubled by the pervading atmosphere. He did not say much, for he felt restrained by external forces. How long would this agony endure? Would there be an end to it, a feeling of redemption to surface after this overwhelming turbulence?

Jon's parents very much wanted to take him away to somewhere familiar. But he was locked away in a place from which he could not escape: the confinement of The Mental Health Act. This had become the pattern of his life, rigid and unforgiving. As time passed, yet more walls were constructed. They towered above Jon's cowering frame. He was left to cry out from the pit of his stomach, his nails tearing into the coarse stone that surrounded him.

Then, one day and out of nowhere, Jon began to offload, with a driven haste, his eyes glaring. They appeared to burn when focused, his body taut as though ready for combat. He spoke so fast that his parents missed a lot of what was said. But they understood the form, if not the content. They hoped that Jon's vocal exorcism would put him on the right road.

This continued for weeks on end as Jon verbally conveyed a myriad of impressions and reflective tales that had shaped his basic character. He would talk with a ferocious energy, covering a wide spectrum of topics, many of which his parents had no knowledge of. Some shocked, others disturbed or illuminated. They began to realise that they had not known their son at all. But now he was opening his heart, they even felt a strange sense of privilege. They needed to hold him, to cherish his new-found affection. For this was the call of their child.

Slowly Jon began to make progress as his medication was reduced and so, in turn, were his side effects. But he was still aware of an emotional blunting and loss of volition. He would walk as though restrained, his limbs weighing him down. When he looked downwards, he could not escape the sight of his butchered arms as they displayed the violence of troubled times. The periods when all that seemed normal were to resort to frenzied mutilation, a release from a sense of vehement self-loathing. During the nocturnal hours Jon would wake, immersed in fear and terror as he fell victim to the nightmares that would endure into day time. These auditory and visual phenomena dominated, leaving Jon shattered and crumpled in the filthy, squalid corners of the time-out room. He felt a shadow of his former self and could not see beyond the emotional scars. During the endless hours, Jon could be seen gazing through the rusting bars that framed the window apertures, longing for feathered wings to capture his dwindling spirits and rise upwards.

LIVES WITHIN A LIFE

Jon hoped that it would not be long before he was transferred to an open ward. His thirst was for freedom, to let the memories fall into the flow of a passing stream. Jon recognised that all of his melancholic wanderings needed to be laid to rest and discarded like an outer skin. His desire was to learn to recognise that this passage in his life had only fortified his resolve and character. In truth, Jon had survived an ordeal that penetrated the essence of his being, and he had returned from a land of extremes. Now he wanted to rebuild his life, to set to work on his visions, words and sounds. He was aware that he possessed an intuitive compassion, directed towards the other patients. All around were those experiencing deepest despair, those who lived with demons tearing into their very souls. Yet internally Jon was coming to realise that he was to be taken from this hell. The blood-stained bars had restrained him for too long. They had to be removed, so that he could be freed to learn from his losses and errors and begin a fresh voyage. Jon had been taken away from the outer world for so long that he now had the impetus to make more of his existence when he returned to relative normality. He did not know the source of his transformation, or its timing, but for the present that was irrelevant. It was now that he must make his escape.

Oh, to be on the run, to rush through the trees, with the wind on his face and to feel intense exhilaration. Jon had been a caged beast, who could never adapt to the confinement of a hospital environment. In his dreams he would jump up into the clouds, his fall cushioned by a profusion of thermals. He had been to hell and back. But when he now gazed across the empty room before him, the chairs and tables were coming to rest. When lost in the realms of richest imagery, Jon was to be taken by a bird of flight to swoop through peak and canyon. It seemed now that it was inevitable that he would escape from the days where there was no light. His soul was to be revitalised, his spirit released. This realisation flooded into Jon's consciousness, leaving him to bathe in the rays that had burned in another time, another manifestation. Now, the angels were calling.

Jon used to inspect his wounds from time to time. Although healed, they had left broad red scars across his arms and neck. Hair had begun to grow where it normally would not, on his wrists, a consequence of the occasions when the lacerations were sown up. The knives had cut deep, tearing the tendons, ripping the veins apart. Jon had come so close to ending his life. There were times he had used cheese graters to ravage his skin, and a lighted cigarette to burn his flesh. He had small craters dotted all over his body. His self-loathing was there for all to see. Inside, however, things were starting to gain momentum, this time in the right direction. Jon would praise God for giving him back what was taken away, and now he was to listen to His commands.

LIVES WITHIN A LIFE

Jon was ushered into the small office that was the venue for the dreaded ward round. He had prepared his case prior to this and planned to ask for discharge. His Section was still in operation and he wanted it to be reviewed. He knew that he would face opposition, for the staff seemed determined to hold him back. Would they hear him?

The consultant in charge was clearly reluctant to let Jon go. The nurses and social workers formed a semi-circle around him and he felt intimidated, as though being fed to lions in the arena. Despite struggling to hide his frustration, Jon perceived a certain lucidity within himself that he tried to convey. Soon he started to become agitated, however, his bodily control rapidly diminishing. He felt that his input was immaterial and that he was smashing his head against a wall. His life was in their hands.

Would these professionals appreciate Jon's needs, his rights and desires, or even find time to listen? Jon wanted to walk out of the office, and onto the street, escaping the law that had incarcerated him for so long. The clinicians were in control, however, and Jon could not overturn their judgment. To him this seemed a time of peculiar imbalance.

As Jon was asked to leave the room, he felt an air of portent. He could almost taste his apprehension. He sat down and lit a cigarette. And then another one. He inhaled deeply and let the smoke stream from his nose. Jon could see faces contorting within the exhalation of nicotine. They danced to an alternative rhythm and then drifted away. He then began to pace whilst holding his head. The anxiety was unbearable, for his actual freedom was at stake. The door opened and Jon was called in. The decision had been made. Jon took a deep breath and clasped the leg of his chair. He was to be moved to an open ward, with a review in a month's time. No argument. No negotiation. His heart sank but what could he do? Jon stood up and walked from the room, without saying a word. His path down the adjacent corridor seemed unusually long. When he reached his room, he slumped onto his bed, his face screwed up. He was beaten. As a consequence of this ruling, Jon had been stripped of any hope of immediate liberty.

He had packed his bags and was ready to be escorted to his new ward. A nurse was to take him and they set off through the grounds. This made quite an impact upon Jon, just to see the green, the splashes of colour, and the graceful fragility of the cedar trees. He listened to the call of the birds and began to think of times when life was less complicated. The sun was blazing and it hurt his eyes, a fact that was exacerbated by the length of time he had been inside. It was glorious to be able to see all that surrounded him. Jon anticipated that one day he would capture these impressions in all manner of mediums. He wanted to evolve as an artist, to continue along a path of discovery. There were patients dotted around, some on benches, others on the grass, most of whom had spent a lifetime here. They were the real lost souls and Jon took solace in the fact that maybe, one day, he would leave. There was still much to endure, however, for this was far from over. The nurse walked in silence, seemingly uninterested. Jon did not care, he was past that. They finally arrived at the open ward and Jon braced himself for life's next chapter.

He was led into a small conservatory, which formed an annex to the main part of the ward. Two patients were sitting, one reading, the other listening to music through headphones. The expanse of glass was immediately welcoming as rays of light shone through, causing angular shadows to break up the wider picture. Jon was introduced to the charge nurse, who appeared friendly and informal. Jon noticed that his eyes looked slightly misty, with a hint of sparkle. Next Jon was shown to his own room, which was basic but comfortable. Soon he set about making it more lived in. On the wall he placed his photograph of David, whose image remained strong and influential. Jon stacked his books on the decidedly ramshackle shelving, with his volumes of art history and photography taking pride of place. He imagined that it was a study where he could immerse himself.

By contrast, the lounge was nicotine-stained,

with the television droning in the corner. There was a pool table, but its felt had been ripped and there was only one cue. Jon noted that the place had been allowed to slip into a state of disrepair, its ambience at odds with its supposed purpose of being a sanctuary. However, it was obviously far more relaxed than the secure unit and it would be home for the immediate future. Jon settled himself in order to build on his theories. He would wake early and walk around the grounds every morning. It was time to make sense of things. At last Jon was free to move unhindered. He could now set his own routine.

After his walk Jon played games with his unconscious. It was all part of an exploration into the realms of seemingly abstract references and the recollection of past experiences. He could be seen sitting, with a packet of cigarettes and cup of coffee, whilst opening doorways into the recesses of his mind. He remained a loner in terms of social contact, and the other patients learned to leave him to himself. Being so private he was not able to converse with ease.

As he sat on the lawn, he attempted to expound his concepts. They were not scientific, but rather a creative release of the subconscious. He had learnt that there was a key to commence this activity. He opened his thoughts, initially into a void. Then he mentally constructed a rectangle in which everything was contained. From this point he would allow an image inside, and it would bounce and collide with the four walls. It could travel at any velocity, and in any direction. Jon compared it to those primitive computer games such as tennis with dots and bats. It worked in the same way. He would concentrate on the initial picture, and then the flurry would commence. All sorts of abstract notions would appear, with no apparent sense of order. Where was this all coming from? Much of what manifested itself was not in any way recognisable. Jon could not even begin to decipher the source of this phenomenon, but that was the fascination: from where did it all originate? Did it belong to Jon's subconscious experience, or was it from another place? He could not fully establish either possibility, but it was his curiosity that drove Jon to try and comprehend it all. Intellectually it tested him, stretching him as he continued with his endeavour. He was formulating a hypothesis regarding the collective sub-conscious. Could it be that at each conception, the mind was filled with a random fragmentation of ancestry? Just as illnesses or disorders were passed down genetically, were these pieces of experience too? Could they be randomly placed into the conscious mind, so influencing strains of behaviour and perception? Could there also be some kind of correlation regarding spiritual matters? Jon felt a great desire to try and uncover essential truths that could form linkages with the whole of the human condition. Jon believed in this although he wished that he could set some parameters, so as to construct a system with which to dissect it all. He wrote down all of his observations, with diagrams and figures. The da Vinci of the ward! He filled his days with many things, this being the start.

Robert Bayley

At mealtimes Jon noticed a man with a shock of silvery grey hair who always sat in the corner. He was immaculately dressed at all times, with a cravat, and a spotted handkerchief in his breast pocket. He possessed fine, almost feline features, with just the slightest suggestion of line or mark to his skin. Visually he was most impressive. Jon had heard on the grapevine that the gentleman was known as 'the doctor.' Jon approached him one teatime and they exchanged pleasantries. The man was obviously very well educated, and spoke in a soft tone. He did, however, appear a little edgy so Jon made a motion to leave. In response to that he was told to stay, and that no offence was taken. Was he really a doctor? Jon could hardly contain his curiosity, and so took the bull by the horns and asked outright. To his complete surprise, the man replied that he was a psychiatrist. What an irony! What could have happened for him to end up here? Jon's mind was accelerating with ever increasing rapidity. Before he could ask the next question, it had been anticipated. The man explained that he was an alcoholic. The demons of drink had ravaged his life to such an extent that he had been struck off by the Medical Council. He had been in private practice for the last ten years of his working life and had drunk progressively more. He could not cope with the sadness and despair in the tales to which he had had to listen. It had all become too much, and the only way he could cope was to hit the bottle. As the drink took a greater hold, he started to lose control of the professional side of his life and was at times aggressive towards clients and increasingly forgetful. This had not escaped the attention of his superiors, and after repeated warnings he was reported and eventually dismissed. He had grown into a monster, controlled by the need to find the next drink. His behaviour worsened, to a point where he despised himself with vehemence. As Jon listened, it dawned on him that this was the first person that he had talked to properly for a long, long time. His parents were the exception, but the doctor was a comparative outsider. Jon's life seemed to be polarised in mood and in terms of social contact.

The doctor had been warned that if he resorted to alcohol again, he would be taking his own life. It was as simple as that. Jon implored him not to, surprising himself with the strength of his call. Jon felt that there was an undeniable bond between them even if it seemed a little premature. He then rose to his feet, went to his room and reflected on all that he had heard.

Like the doctor, Jon had been given another chance. The memory of what had occurred that fateful day in Amsterdam was never to leave him. But such was his despair, Jon had seen no other way. A wall had crashed down on top of him as any semblance of order had been stripped from his mind. He recalled the view from the skylight in his apartment where he was lost in romantic escapism. Jon had worked hard to bring all his memories into context. Now however, he endeavoured to progress, to escape the compulsion to mutilate. He had not played his instruments for a long time now, nor filled a canvas with his bloody images and it left a void. All of his life Jon had been under attack, from his conception to the present, aching day. The only prospect that held it all together was his prophecy of a creative fusion in which his spiritual rays would envelop and heal the afflicted. For the moment there was a battle in the skies, its clouds streaked in red, casting a shadow on the pitiful existence of those below. Jon envisaged his own image standing tall, lit from above. He could find solace in the fortress of his heart. It was full of goodness, the demons cast out.

Jon and the doctor used to meet in the music room most evenings. Tonight was one of those occasions. On the turntable was some wild jazz composition and the two of them were listening in silence. Strains of muted trumpet and alto saxophone could be heard, driving the beat. The doctor asked Jon what message the sounds conveyed to him. Could he imagine colours and pictures, was there any narrative? In response Jon felt that the flood gates were opening, allowing his creative juices to flow in glorious abundance. He could sense all the colours and tones, all the gradations of line and form. Jon was experiencing a profusion of intensification. There was nothing to contain it.

These conceptual explorations were a source of great pleasure to this unlikely pair. They both considered that they shared an intellectual passion for the arts and were able to reciprocally bounce ideas from one to the other. The imagery was profound, and their dialogue stimulating. Jon and the doctor had discovered a certain linkage between them that was rare and, as a consequence, was to be treasured. Just as importantly, they understood the despair of mental suffering and were able, by way of sympathetic compassion, to help each other find a path through their private hell. As they faced the day, over coffee and cigarettes, there now seemed to be a bit of brightness. This progression was of great value and their conversations activated the mind, thus providing distraction from those distortions that cruelly brought pain to the essence of their being. They had found friendship.

As though inspired, Jon proceeded to speak of the day when everything had been magical. He was a young boy, careering across the parkland. He remembered the balloons, the play and the exuberance that afternoon exuded. Everything was perfect, and Jon had never wanted it to end. It was all so vivid now. If only he could transport himself back to times of such happiness, when innocence prevailed. Jon's memories flowed with precise detail. He explained the transition from that time to the war zone that was today's reality. The doctor listened patiently. He was becoming a faithful companion.

As the music continued to play, the pair took to writing verse to accompany it according to the mood of the piece, or telling stories, based on truth or fantasy. Sometimes a bit of both. This was possibly the beginning of great works! To Jon, a feeling of excitement was returning. A mixture of literary semantics and choral crescendo was pouring forth, in multitude and in the form of creative adventure. As they rode on the crest of the wave, Jon noticed that in the far corner there was a decrepit piano, which had seen better days. Jon sat on the stool and opened the lid. He had explained to the doctor how long it had been since he had last played an instrument. With apprehension he placed his hands on the keys. He hit a chord, and it was drenched in glorious reverberation. The action of the piano was beautifully light and Jon began to improvise. He would first wait to hear the sounds internally and then transpose them into tangible realms. Before long Jon had become reacquainted with the keyboard, and it felt wonderful. The doctor congratulated him, recognising his gift.

These times helped Jon to rejuvenate his passion for the arts. From those opening chords and verse, he gained enthusiasm. It was as though Jon was entering a whole new world, a place that accorded with his enthusiastic sense of purpose. He was relearning the art of expression whilst losing himself in worlds where there are no boundaries, no limitations. This had been provoked by the touch of ivory keys on the skin. The doctor had eased open the door. However, Jon was now aware of a pervading intensity when he was with the doctor that left him feeling uneasy. Initially he was unable to pinpoint the exact cause of this wariness. He put it down as an intuitive feeling that would explain itself in time. The nature of their closeness was altering and as a consequence, Jon started to withdraw and restrict his contact a little. There were times when Jon could feel the heat of an intense gaze, aimed at him, leaving him unable to respond. The doctor was transforming into some needy youth, lost in the ardour of teenage passion. As much as Jon could ascertain, he had not laid down any seed of encouragement. So what was the source? Was this all some bizarre manifestation of his inherent paranoia, Jon opined internally? As time passed by, this notion was rejected as Jon could sense an air that was somewhat inappropriate, misplaced even. Jon felt a physical presence from the doctor that he could not reciprocate, so that their evenings of music appreciation became more and more sporadic as did normal conversation. What had been special now seemed jaded. In response the doctor appeared increasingly tortured and pained. Any explanation remained elusive.

Eventually, the doctor confronted Jon, explaining that he wanted to provide him with everything that was lacking in his own life, elements such as security and stability. He wanted to offer a sense of care and balance. But from this root his concern had become a painful affection and he apologised for any pressure he might have exerted. He articulated a deep sense of longing; their relationship seemed to be entering another sphere. But this area did not appeal to Jon. It conjured up feelings of uncertainty and dependency, which he had to reject. What had happened to this unlikely pair? Jon needed to have time to himself, to be alone.

Jon could not cope with what had been expressed by the doctor and he was considering breaking off any contact with him. He felt no malice, but wanted rather to move away from the burning flame of desire. In a sense he wanted to protect the doctor but was aware that he would miss their friendship as the doctor had always been there for him, had never judged him and had consistently supported him. Jon had felt able to convey his deepest thoughts, his fears and weaknesses. Jon decided to speak to the doctor. He found him by the record player, which had become their meeting place. Jon began to explain that it was best for them to end their friendship as it had become too complex and entwined with misplaced passion. Jon said that he would always care for him, but that it was now appropriate for them to go their separate ways in order to provide a guard for the doctor's powerful feelings. He then turned and left.

Inside what was now a hollow room the doctor started to sob, quivering from head to foot for he knew the affair was over. Now he needed Jon more than ever.

A while later Jon passed the music room and heard the sound of crying between the crackle of old vinyl. He recognised the wail and scream but closed the door to his heart and returned to his room. That was the last time he saw the doctor. Only the new dawn would reveal the truth.

The next day Jon was woken early as usual by

the nurses. His limbs felt heavy as he rose from his slumber. But immediately it became apparent that it was not a normal day. There was a palpable sense of urgency. The nurses asked what had happened between him and the doctor the previous evening. Jon began to explain the course of events, remembering the discord, but then stopped and asked what was wrong. They replied that the doctor had not returned to the ward and was missing. He had been out all night. Jon's heart began to race and he was soon in a state of blind panic. He was told to stay on the ward whilst the grounds were scoured. There was nothing he could do, just sit tight.

Paradoxically Jon felt he needed a stiff drink to calm his nerves. How ridiculous that was! He hoped that before long he would see the doctor's face, for him to be found, unharmed. The waiting was unbearable. Jon was unable to distract himself as all manner of ghastly possibilities shot through his head. He was overwhelmed by sheer anxiety. The minutes turned into hours, with no report, no news of the doctor's fate. Jon slipped down a wall to support his weary frame and crouched, holding his head. He squeezed his eyes shut. Eventually the searchers returned, their faces hidden. Jon knew instantly that his darkest fears had been realised. He approached the charge nurse, to hear the worst. He was told that the doctor was dead. His corpse had been found, sprawled beside the cedar tree. Beside him was his Remy Martin, and in his hand a piece of Jon's verse.

At the foot of the page was the doctor's

declaration of love for Jon. He had adored him, and realised that his love would never be shared. As a consequence the doctor had died by his own hand.

Jon howled and cried, totally absorbed by loss, his sense of guilt all consuming.

Jon became acutely withdrawn and lived in almost constant silence for several months. He could not bring himself to communicate readily. The doctor was gone now and Jon prayed for his soul. If only he could have anticipated the doctor's demise. The depth of his grief cut to the quick, tearing his emotions apart. Jon thought of the times shared and the alcohol that had wiped it all away. It was a cruel end to a flawed existence. The death turned out to be a symbol of great sacrifice. Perhaps Jon had taken the most precious part of him by rejecting his affection. The doctor had listened to his own darker thoughts, which were exacerbated by the toxicity of drink. He had lost charge of his body and mind. His relationship with Jon initially began to fill the chasm left when his vocation was stripped from him. This had become obsessive, to the point that the doctor had become convinced that they would fall into each other's arms. Jon however, was attracted to his kindliness and intellect, but that was all. As Jon viewed the cedar tree from a distance, he realised that this whole affair had been a tale of unrequited love. A feeling of unavoidable remorse overwhelmed him and he did not know where to turn.

The cliche of the never ending tunnel had never felt so accurate. Jon felt that he was being propelled into the more destructive recesses of his mind. Places where he felt tempted to release his pain by way of self mutilation. He was longing for solutions, but when he perceived that they were approaching, he was thrust back into the psychotic dreams of the stormy night time. As Jon gazed at the moon he could hear the howls of emaciated wolves and he could see his own battle streaked in blood on the surrounding hill tops. This torture would linger on and on, unless Jon would be able to transform his outlook and become defiant.

Jon called out to the heavens for an escape from this descending spiral. He wanted to awaken in that elusive land where calm prevailed. His desire was to transcend to the magical times, where the spectrum of glistening light spread far. Jon had reached a point where transition was imperative, to use experience as a manifestation of depth and resilience.

As time passed, Jon began to feel a little easier but progress was painfully slow. He could not eradicate the guilt that dominated his conscious thoughts. All he could do was pray that the doctor was at peace. Maybe he would never know, but he longed to have some indication and faith that the storm was over. Many images lingered, some more abstract, others more directly symbolic of the doctor's desperate expression. Jon was to reflect on his emotions as they took the form of auditory phenomena. These voices came from all directions and would increase in their vehemence until they penetrated the central part of Jon's psyche. They would comment and refer to memories and impressions from days past to a degree of obsession. From this violent and intense base Jon intended to convert his negative energy into the domain of positivity.

Jon's routine had started to get back to normal. He hoped that it would not be long before he left the hospital. It would not come a moment too soon. An inherent part of his recovery was to be only reliant on his own resources, even if that necessitated becoming a loner again. Jon used to walk to town some days, buy music, have a coffee, absorb the activity. But he was always alone. In his room he produced pencil studies of his immediate environment, for he was overwhelmed by inspiration. Pieces of paper were strewn over the floor as creativity began to warm the blood in his veins. Jon's loss was mysteriously provoking him to reflect more and form imagery that encapsulated the grief.

His parents continued to visit but little was said; there was a sparseness of communication. In contrast to more distant times, Jon did realise that they were around and that was the most important element. His parents regarded Jon as a lost soul.

LIVES WITHIN A LIFE

They longed for the day when they could take him away, to hold him in their arms.

Despite Jon's current state of mind, the turn of the next corner would bring more than he could ever imagine. It would turn out to be the most influential and uplifting part of his life.

Jon was seated in the conservatory, looking aimlessly out of the window. He was dreaming of more contented climes, to take him away from these wild, meandering passages. He could see the smoking lounge through the open door, allowing the stench of cigarettes to drift in. Jon could hear the other patients in discussion, interspersed with the occasional burst of laughter. It was just a normal day. Or so he thought. His stomach was crying out for food, and Jon was counting the minutes until dinner time. There were so many voids to try and fill. Jon considered it to be faintly ridiculous to mark out the day by mealtimes, but that was part of his way of surviving the regime, of attempting to transcend the boredom and lack of external stimulation. Jon was aware that he must try to avoid becoming a vegetable himself. The medicine did not help either, even if it had been reduced since the days when he spent most of his time restrained under lock and key. He was full of anger and frustration and he longed for a guiding light, to show him the right path. Jon could sense that an air of desperation was to be laid to rest.

It was then that he saw her. In an armchair

facing the conservatory was the most captivatingly beautiful woman. It was as though she had suddenly appeared out of nowhere, like a magician's illusion. Jon could not take his eyes off her, for he even considered that she might indeed be an apparition. Was this all a trick of the mind? An oasis in the endless, rolling dunes? No, she was as real as flesh and bone.

Jon went to sit on a sofa in the other room, positioning himself so that she could not register his attention. He wanted to observe her undisturbed whilst wondering whether her personality matched her wondrous looks. Jon sensed that there was no disparity. This longing caused Jon to feel that the world was becoming alive again and he wanted this vibrancy to grow in profusion. To Jon, she had no flaws; her defined features, her deep auburn hair and the most startling brown eyes were appreciated. Her skin was golden and unblemished, her hands so anatomically delicate. As she opened her mouth, her teeth shone, and were perfectly formed. Jon could sense a lightness and delicacy in her disposition. He could also perceive a sharp intellect and wit with which to enthral. Jon was utterly mesmerised.

As he lowered his gaze, he saw bandages covering her wrists and noticed that her posture was almost apologetic. What had happened to her? Jon reflected that mental despair can afflict us all. Inside he was stirring, wanting to vocalise, to communicate. It was as if there had always been a space inside for her. He focused on her eyes again, and they twinkled like precious stones. Jon felt that she would become the most treasured person in his world, and he would never leave her side. His heart overflowed and now he must connect with her. She was so beautiful.

Over the next week or so, Jon tried to be patient. He could see that the object of his desire was deeply troubled, yet he wanted to speak to her and for her to respond. Paradoxically he was full of words, but he did not know what to say. She isolated herself and Jon could relate to that, for in the past he had done the same. He wanted to reach out to her, but was so apprehensive that he never quite made it. He would retreat to his room and write poetry, which was full of passion and fire. He would illustrate the verse with oil pastels, creating the most romantic of images. Would he ever be able to profess his love? Jon wanted to come across as self-assured and not appear a fool. He knew that he was genuine and true, but would she recognise these qualities? There were instances when he had come close to speaking, and then the moment would pass. Jon tried to get a grip on his emotions, to channel the ardour. She was the woman of his dreams, to whom he had not said a single word. He had fallen in love and he knew he had to act before she vanished from his life. Jon could sense the clock ticking.

From time to time Jon would notice her smiling, which he saw as a positive sign. He had even managed to say the occasional hello, to which she had replied, but with hesitation. At one time she had looked straight into his eyes, causing him to tremble without control. Now he knew the opportunity had come.

Jon found her alone in the music room. He had picked his moment. He stood outside the door for what seemed a painfully long while and then entered. Immediately there was a palpable sense of anticipation in the air. This seemed to equate with the frightening magnification of Jon's emotional state. He sat down carefully and opened his mouth, but nothing came out. He looked around uneasily and then began to stare at the floor. The awkward pair then tried to introduce themselves at exactly the same time! This was amusing to them both and they laughed, nervously.

It transpired that her name was Sarah and Jon was eager to learn more about her. He could not distance himself from feelings of endearment, but he tried not to convey too much intrigue as he did not want to overwhelm her. Suddenly she jumped to her feet, gave a mumbled apology and left the room. Jon did not know whether he had contributed to this unexpected action; was it because he was too overbearing, he asked himself? He really had no idea. Anyway, he felt rotten. He remained in the room and lit cigarette after cigarette. Why was this happening, he wondered?

Jon missed his next meal as he had no appetite. He felt physically ill; this was the sickness of love. He was overwhelmed by the sweats, his head and heart pounding. He could think of nothing else or show any interest in anything, apart from his beloved Sarah.

A few hours had passed and as Jon walked up one of the endless corridors, he caught sight of Sarah at the other end. He called after her and, to his amazement, she stopped and turned to face him. He proceeded to tell her of the extent of his extravagant passion, as he could contain it no longer. Oh, the relief he experienced as he poured forth with his expression of purest adoration! She fell into his arms, holding him tight. Initially she had not realised the extent of his feelings, but she would reciprocate it all. They grabbed each other's hands and ran to the grass outside.

They sat beneath the cedar tree where the doctor had passed away and Jon explained how he had been immersed in grief. The more he talked of it, the less disturbing the memories became. Sarah seemed to understand it all. Jon felt that he had always known her. She explained that she had run from the music room as she could not control her impulses. She had wanted him right from the start, but never had the confidence to express or show her desires. Jon displayed a sensitive compassion to what Sarah had revealed and then held her, his tears flowing.

They felt they shared a common bond, as though they had the same blood; from that day they would be complete. From beneath the trees they lost all count of time. Nightfall came as they lay together, sometimes in silence, at other times full of vocal interplay. They wanted to walk out of the gates of the institution and say goodbye to the past. Together they would face the tomorrows, and resolve any trials and tribulations. This was how Jon wanted to live his life, not alone, as his empty years had dictated. Now he could express all his longing, with unprecedented conviction and without fear.

Jon and Sarah spent almost every waking hour together. They dreamed of life outside the asylum, where liberty would allow hope and opportunities to evolve. The times under the cedar tree would prove the most poignant. Its trunk was theirs, and the symbolic recounting of Jon's nightmares and their subsequent closure helped transform the guilt he felt over the doctor.

Sarah was to be pivotal in turning Jon around and opening him up, for he had become very preoccupied by the demons he experienced. Jon now felt safe and loved. The two used to walk together, speaking of every subject and every feeling. They felt that they had been brought together by forces greater than themselves.

It transpired that Sarah had become ill after flirting with amphetamines, unaware of the potential consequences. She had started to indulge herself when part of a rebellious group at school. After education had finished, the drug filled the empty days when she was on the dole and directionless. Her parents were consumed by work since they owned their own business. Her brother was at university, and was always distant and unapproachable. He was an academic, and was now studying for a doctorate in psychology. Sarah had always considered herself inferior to him, and this was exacerbated by her lack of contact with her parents. The drugs seemed to offer a way out. The reality was that it had become more ominous than mere flirtation. It had taken hold of her mind and body and Sarah became increasingly paranoid. It coloured her complete perception of life and in the end she had attempted suicide. She had sunk into deepest despair.

It was an existence that was now coming to a conclusion. Sarah realised that with Jon's help she could end her dependency. The people she had mixed with were not even companions; their only concern was for the drug. They had all dropped out of society and had no intention of returning to it. Ironically, Sarah's attempt to take her own life had saved her. At times she would speak to Jon about the group she had been with, wondering if they had survived. She would never find out.

Sarah's parents could not accept what had happened to their daughter. All they could do was condemn it, without even trying to understand. The resentment between them was considerable. But she no longer seemed to care. Her relationship with Jon was what really mattered. Jon's parents took to Sarah straight away, despite their instinctive protectiveness. She seemed so buoyant, forward-thinking and practical. And Jon's obvious happiness was infectious. In all aspects the couple had made provision for each other and were complete.

It would not be long before Jon and Sarah were to leave the place that had taken so much and in turn given back, by way of their meeting each other. They began to plan for life beyond the harsh realities of incarceration and they anticipated that the world could stand against them. The days had been long, the months dragging by. Jon's liberty had been removed, supposedly to treat his distress. It had caused regression as the bars had imprisoned him, with spontaneity constrained. Jon had been punished by oppressive behaviour programmes which denied individuality and were marked by rigidity. He yearned to feel the pulse of free thinking and creativity and to identify with concepts with which to express himself.

Now there had been a metamorphosis within Jon's view of life, as he had found his mate. His friendship with Sarah was cemented by a bond which was both elastic and constant. On the few occasions when Jon was alone, he craved for Sarah. It was not a mark of obsession, rather an expression of need. She possessed that elusive empathy. Matters did not need to be endlessly explained for she was quick to understand, whatever the theme.

Jon continued to write, and embellish his prose with drawings, building upon his illustrative technique. When he looked above and into the skies, he could see facets of Sarah's gemlike face. She would beam down, releasing the lines on his brow like the rays of the sun. He could also see reminders of her in the flowers by the borders of sinewy paths, as they evolved, displaying their timeless beauty. Jon would pick the vibrantly coloured daffodils, arrange them and bring them as gifts. He carved pieces of wood into the softest of shapes, taking Sarah's form as his inspiration. Jon had taken her hand, giving everything of himself, as he proclaimed his love without conditions or rules. There had been an expansion of Jon's vision, his sense of purpose more clearly defined. The negative elements that had brought despair had now been transformed beyond the wildest of dreams. The battlements that had previously enclosed were now left smouldering in the dust.

Outside, the skies were alive with energy, as lightning struck, fragmenting and slicing through the darkness, the thunder rolling. The rain was coming down in relentless torrents, beating savagely against the streaky window panes. This imagery reminded Jon of his childhood, when he would find solace behind the settee as the storm battered the earth below it. But now Sarah was with him, holding and gently kissing his forehead. Everything that had provoked fear and consternation would now be healed and resolved completely. A cocoon in which to protect, Jon stayed inside his love until the morning, as he could not bear to let her go. He would never relinquish his hold, for they were to be together forever.

CHAPTER FOUR - LOVE

Jon and Sarah were in the Lake District for a well-earned break. It was during the warmest of summer times and the sun was blazing, the sky imbued in rich azure. The pair had rented a small cottage for their retreat from the madding metropolis and they were surrounded by forest and pasture. The sound of the nearby sheep greeted them every morning, as the cacophony of the city had been replaced by dulcet tones to soothe the weary soul. Sometimes they woke at dawn, if only to appreciate the freshness and beauty of their location. Jon sat with his sketch pad and attempted to document the moods and impressions that encompassed him. There was always a bowl of fresh fruit on the patio, along with fresh coffee and its particular aroma, with packs of tobacco to indulge the desire for nicotine. Jon had also brought his camera and lenses, to capture the enormity of the scenery. His receptors were working over-time for there was much to appreciate and to savour. From indoors, free-form jazz emanated from the stereo, rebounding against the walls and passages. For them both, this was the sweetest of times.

During the day Jon and Sarah took to the hills and mountains, with backpacks containing provisions and explored the peaks and valleys. From the summits they would look over the unfolding landscape, in deserved states of exhaustion! Jon recorded the myriad of images onto film, not only for posterity, but also to help him form the basis of greater works when they returned home, on board and canvas. He also remained dedicated to his verse, describing his relationship with Sarah, and now there were books full of his words for her.

When in heightened and prolific creative states, Jon's paint brush would dance over the paper, commencing with washes and subsequently adorned with fine detail. When using the more painterly medium of oils, Jon built up uneven, textural layers that equated with the unpredictable biochemical makeup of his own vulnerable brain. He also kept journals, from day to day. These would help him to formulate ideas and to recall events and experiences with precision. There were occasions when Jon was quite overwhelmed by all that he had assimilated, especially the intensity and power. Jon would dream of periods when he could ease this sense of vehemence and rejuvenate his jaded bones. However, his outlook was now rooted in positive realms, which was a marked and welcome contrast.

Jon felt he could view the world from the mountain tops and plunge into the lakes below. Rock formations framed the vista and Jon allowed his vision to expand, absorbing the glory and splendour of this flawed but beautiful planet. Sarah stood beside him and she shared the same perspective, such was her intuition. She was always full of energy and this influenced Jon, for now he had a spring in his step. The pair would rush down from the summits, slipping and sliding, sporting the broadest of grins. They had attained a tangible certainty and triumph which they could not contain.

In the evenings they would drink a little wine, prepare food together and enjoy each other's company. Their conversation was animated and the subject matter they covered was vast. Sarah was an avid reader and over the years she had taken in many of the classic icons of literature, from the philosophy of the ancient Greeks, to the contemporary masters. To hear her recount fine details enthralled Jon, his interest maintained and constant. During these literary excursions a farm house cat had taken to wandering in at supper time, looking for scraps. It would sit staring at Sarah, as though absorbing her every move. It would then follow them into the sitting room and curl up on Jon's chest, snug in his sweater.

This really was the most idyllic place to reside, and Jon and Sarah wished they could stay forever. So, when they returned home, Jon was eager to start transposing his sketches and photographs onto canvas, forming a pictorial record of their experience in The Lakes. Some of these would be between six to eight feet tall and they were a fitting monument to their stay. But there was always the next time to look forward to, the continuation of the adventure into the real world, beyond the rusting gates of institutional care. This loving pair were in control of their destiny now, they could decide the course of their existence and they immersed themselves in the glow. The currents above carried their dreams to horizons new. The anticipation was intense.

Jon and Sarah rented a small house on the

edge of town. It had been constructed in the Victorian era and possessed a certain quaint charm. The brick work had been left untouched, only the roof tiles had been replaced in recent years and the paintwork reapplied. Flashes of vibrant colour adorned the frontage, by way of drooping fuschia and delicate rose. There was much to admire for this dwelling was aesthetically most pleasing. Jon's parents were only ten minutes' walk away and Jon and Sarah would often visit them, either for a meal or morning coffee. In return for their kindness, Jon would help with the gardening, planting herbs and flowers. This work was a positive discipline to which Jon reacted favourably. There were always parts of the garden that required attention, an ongoing project. There was now a dog in the family, which had been rehomed after being maltreated during his formative years. He had been named Duke, after Duke Ellington, the jazz musician, and was full of bounce and enthusiasm. He was a scruffy mongrel, his coat a mish-mash of shades of brown, ginger and white. Jon would take him for long walks, out into the fields, and let him bound and chase after rabbit and hare. But when Duke had had enough, he would just lie down and refuse to get up. He needed a rest, and that was it. No argument. This would always make Jon laugh.

At home, Jon had converted the loft into what he called the "fusion" room. Fusion referred to the nucleus of his creative exploration, encompassing imagery, literature and sound. Rather like Amsterdam, this was all located within a central area but within a real home this time. Inside the room Jon had arranged his recording equipment, along with his basses and guitars and a synthesiser with which to create sounds. These elements were the tools with which to turn the sounds that would never leave him, into reality. During the darkest hours, in the midst of thunder and storm, Jon would hold onto those strains of lyrical, modal scales and aching, diminished chords; running to the "fusion" room in the middle of the night, if only to capitalise on and capture that elusive melody. There he had formed a library of harmony, verse and rhythm. There was also plenty of room to paint, with unused canvases leaning against the walls, ready to be covered with pigment, streaked across every fibre, forming abstract images. Jon regarded the actual process of initial conceptualisation leading to the application of various media, one of constant fascination. Just as the music would lead and enthral, so too would the magical quality of building images from any source, thus allowing the observer to be affected.

In the far corner was a writing desk, upon which sat a word processor which Jon used to collate his journals and verse. He was certainly a technophobe but regarded his computer as a necessary evil. It helped him keep all his ideas and reflections in immaculate order, for Jon had real pride in his work as well as his location and its ambience. He would also carve and sculpt, producing caricatures which refined his observational skills. They were his source of amusement and the sculptures conveyed his love for the human form. The oil paintings were both his window and mirror. He was now laying the quintessential foundations for the projection of his artistic dreams. He had thought of the domes and peaks of his journey many times over the years, and they did not lose their intensity. He had continued to work, initially sourced from the roots of inspiration and from there to the pinnacle of achievement. All previous psychotherapeutic advice to avoid extremes was being thrown to the wind, for any immersion in the passion of improvisation carried risk. This could only contribute to a state of stimulus and excitement.

All the walls of the house were adorned with Jon's prints, drawings and paintings. Sarah was proud of him and his achievements. In a personal sense, her desires for oblivion had retreated and she felt whole now, her life as she had always wanted it. There seemed to be an inherent stability to her existence, but also a contentment that she had never previously experienced. There was a warmth deep inside. Jon had not had a relapse for over a year now, and Sarah prayed that it would continue that way. They had managed to survive the most brutal of regimes, but their chance meeting made sense of it all. The institution had been the most desolate of places, where hope was left to dissipate into the endless corridors, where screams could be heard, hollering in savage torment. The memories of time-out confinement were etched on the inner mind as inextricably as the scars on the flesh. It had taken a lot of adjustment to deal with life without constraint and constant, intimidating observation.

Jon and Sarah needed time to adjust and to understand the new roles they found themselves in. They, particularly Jon, had become institutionalised. He had been in a place where many of the day-to-day responsibilities that were in the domain of relative normality had been taken away. Now, decisions had to be made in all aspects of life and to Jon this meant structuring the day so that there were disciplines to adhere to and in turn, provide balance. At times it was an immense struggle, and he wanted to cave in, to give in to the pressure in his head. Sarah, however, was always there to encourage him and to break the pattern of potential decline, for it must not become ingrained. The positive must override and for this stable period it did.

Jon continued to work on his musical equations, taking samples of different sounds and then reassembling them. He would sample ethnic drums, sinewy bass lines, aching rumbles and orchestral strings which he had always favoured and add them to his already considerable arsenal of auditory stimulus. He was concerned with constructing collages and sweeps of sound, taking in all aspects of modulation and timbre. Sometimes Jon would see all this interaction as though a hologram, forever changing according to one's viewpoint. It was all so dense and rich, yet simultaneously illuminating.

Jon had become interested in the natural occurrence of texture and would spend days searching for different examples. Bark, stone, grain, he juxtaposed them all. When their pattern was captured on film, their collective tonality was mesmerising to this obsessive artist. He had begun to realise his purpose, but there was much more to expose and it would all be revealed in a cataclysmic finale.

The house was full of this vibrancy, which Jon's parents picked up on when they visited. To them it was a time of expectancy and excitement. Their son was achieving so much, they could hardly believe it. Especially when they cast their minds back to the days of the residency in Amsterdam and ensuing hospitalisation. They all enjoyed simple things; sitting in the garden during summer evenings, toasting around the fire during the bleaker months. Sometimes their laughter would resound into the small hours, to the extent that their sides ached! But it was the fact that they were now really close that meant the most. Life seemed whole; a real transformation.

Jon had taken to walking Duke every day now which was a good routine. The dog had become a good and loyal friend. This was displayed when Jon entered his parents' house. The dog would career down the stairs and jump right up to him, his paws reaching up to Jon's shoulders. Jon considered himself to be his master, such was their increasingly inseparable relationship. The patterns of exercise relieved Jon's father of any sense of responsibility as he suffered from arthritis and so was unable now to walk Duke properly. Jon would take the dog all over town, across the undulating turf of the public parks and then explore the meandering routes that made up the country lanes. During these times, Jon had begun to talk to Duke and he would look up with affection as Jon spoke. His tail was always wagging, his eyes soft and welcoming. When they reached the point of weariness the two would lie down in the fields as Duke panted for breath. Jon had taken to resting on Duke's belly and then to gazing at the transient nature of the cloud formations above. Jon lost his thoughts in a curious dream-like reality and he imagined that he was drifting into the heavens. He visualised a capsule that had descended to this earth to capture and contain his fears; a spiritual armour with which to protect him from secular attack.

This routine would take place every day, usually in the late afternoon. The pair would return to the house, both exhausted after their jaunt. As time passed by, Sarah was becoming concerned for Jon. Because she could not be specific as to the source of her anxiety, she did not broach the subject. Despite attempts to distract herself, she was unable to distance herself from a sense of impending dread. Sarah thought that Jon was possibly starting to lose control of his mind again. She became very fearful as she contemplated the possibility. It would be savagely cruel to strip away all that had been achieved. For the moment she would just watch from the sidelines and pick up any peculiarities. For she would be the one to see them first, such were her powers of perception.

During the night Jon would appear more and more fitful, but with no recollection of these experiences in the morning. He woke covered in a cold sweat, his body trembling without control. Tears streamed down his cheeks, his mouth barely able to form coherent words, Jon was screaming in a nocturnal hell. Was this the start of the night terrors that Jon had experienced when in the institution? It seemed a possibility to Sarah as she held him, praying for a cleansing from any demons that were attempting to corrupt Jon's soul. She begged for him to be spared.

Jon and Sarah had evolved together like the seamless progression of incoming waves. The home that they had made for themselves was in their personal style and as a consequence was an integral part of them. Their abode was more than mere bricks and mortar, for it conveyed the way the foundations of their relationship were secure and absolute. In their own way the two were using the benefit of many years of mental challenges to aid the removal of suffering. Jon was a dreamer, but he retained a certain resolve to confront the contorted and grotesque. He was also supremely capable of capturing emotive reflections on the rhythms of this strange life. By his side was Sarah, who was an individual who pieced lives back together. She showed an empathy with those individuals who had everything stripped from them, including their faith and their dignity.

Within Jon's increasingly fragile mind, he now perceived that he was living on his own little island, fishing for provisions. As he viewed his scrawny and emaciated frame, those scars symbolising the bleakest times had turned a deep crimson, their pattern like a busy map. He could feel the warmth of Sarah's breath on his neck and he turned to face her, as she crouched down, building the fire. The ocean was lapping up onto the shore, leaving its mark on the shifting sands. As hours passed into days, elements became more unsettled, just as there was always the threat of derangement in the volatile parts of the mind. Jon yearned to discover a place in which to hide from demonic penetration. He felt the desire to piece together some improvised shelter, within which his skin could lie by Sarah's golden flesh. But as he looked skywards, all Jon could see were knives falling to the ground like atmospheric tears. Maybe they had always been lurking ominously, but now they were rapidly approaching. As Jon immersed himself in deepest thought, he surmised that the key lay with Duke.

Jon believed that there were secret codes being left in Duke's urine. Each time he relieved himself against a lamp post, strains of information were dispensed in microscopic scale, all of which referred to Jon's thoughts and experiences. Now the dog would project this data towards menacing forces, for there was a conspiracy proliferating. When Jon was asleep he dreamt of Duke being slaughtered, like an animal in the abattoir. This turned out to be the reason for Jon's disturbed sleep patterns, which so worried Sarah. A manifestation of dread, of loss, all encapsulated in a brutal, extreme manner. Duke had been a companion who refrained from judgement and was consistent in his behaviour at all times. But would his love for his master remain when Jon plunged into a period of wild and uncontrollable mania? For this strained and heightened activity affected Jon dramatically.

It all started with the lamp posts, like a seed that had been planted and allowed to multiply. But it swiftly catapulted Jon into a paranoiac world. This acceleration was shocking to the observers that made up Jon's family. These members were significant for different reasons however, for Jon believed that they were being manipulated by the Devil, and that the conspiratorial plot was tightening. By the dispersion of his fluids, fragments of accumulated information were being placed by Duke in an extremely confusing way and Jon was growing increasingly wary of him. But such was his love and affection for this previously trustworthy hound, Jon did not want to leave him. Here was the existence of contradictions and inconsistencies that led Jon down a florid and precarious path. Although more intermittently, Jon continued to converse with Duke, and to hear his projections. But as he stroked his fur, there appeared to be electrical surges passing through him. Jon would feel an energy rush that reached every extremity with an undeniable potency. Jon felt a vigour and dynamism that overwhelmed him, but all the messages he received were muddled; on one hand the dog was as faithful as ever and on the other, he was embroiled in persecutory complexity. But what was the root of these bodily upsurges? Duke did not answer, but the severity of the sensations endured.

One day it all came to a head. Jon and Duke

were in their local park and Jon stepped down to fix Duke's lead. They had completed a long walk, incorporating many areas lined with foliage and tracks twisting like vast, elongated serpents. As they continued with their wanderings, Jon had been experiencing the most penetrative of voices and his anxiety levels were rising. He surveyed the immediate vicinity and felt that he was going to faint. In endeavouring to resist this sensation, Jon fell to his knees. He was a crumpled wreck on the ground and Duke approached with an uncharacteristic air of trepidation. To his utter surprise, Jon then heard the call of the saxophonist from the band and instinctively turned to reply. As he did, all he could see was the musician's face, his whole body removed. He proceeded to float in and out of Jon's field of vision and then disappeared. This apparition was fleeting, but profound. It marked a part of Jon's history, a time of great creativity and also suffering. Now there seemed to be the start of another passage of mental decay.

Jon came over with a chill, looked down to his feet and ran. Duke was right by his side and they stormed down the roads and streets until they arrived home. In terms of distance, they had covered three or four miles, but in their energised state it had seemed more like a hundred yards. Man and beast then crashed through the front door, Jon covered in streams of sweat and Duke panting vigorously. Sarah was with Jon's parents and they ran into the hallway, immediately sensing Jon's distress. The family were all anxious to know what had happened. Jon was about to reply, when his old psychiatrist appeared before him and commanded him to say nothing. He proceeded to tell him that the authorities were looking for evidence to put him away, to send him back to the institution. The vision of the clinician was photographic in its vividness, and the instruction was deemed by Jon to be absolute. Like the saxophonist, he then disappeared into a hopeless void.

Jon was totally disorientated but could not give voice to his fears. He felt that he was held in an emotional straight jacket, a restraining device that denied him self-expression. He had been captured by a speeding rollercoaster, from which he could not escape. The visions were now projected in profusion and soon the spirit of the doctor who died by his own hand became visible. He was to prepare Jon for some bad news: a revelation that would have far-reaching consequences.

He told Jon that Sarah had been having an affair and had grown to despise him. Jon screamed out in terror, reaching down into the bowels of hell. How could she have done this, he cried? Jon bellowed at Sarah, attacking her with a torrent of abuse. Jon wanted her to leave, never to return. He was totally poisoned by this deception, for he could not distinguish truth from crazed deceit. Sarah had no idea what was going on and began to sob uncontrollably. She was frightened not only by the content of the abuse, but also by its ferocity. Jon then took to running up and down the stairs, whilst continuing to hurl insults. Loyal as ever, Duke followed him, wherever he went. Jon would go from one room to the next, with no apparent purpose. Within his brain all of those misunderstood biochemicals were driving this manic individual into an acute episode of hyper-activity. The family tried to control him but when they approached him they were met with a flurry of fists. Jon caught his father in the eye, drawing blood. Sarah was imploring him to stop, frantic in her worry. Jon then sat down, his feet kicking back and forth. The cushions became alive and would send out orders, compelling Jon to punch his own face, howling as he did. He was behaving like a caged, haunted animal, with no chance of release.

Jon's parents had no idea what to do. Sarah was beginning to withdraw into her inner shell, for she could not cope with what she was witnessing. The family did not want to call the doctor, else they would risk losing him all over again. In desperation his mother locked the doors and hid the keys in an inner pocket. At least they could try and contain the situation and attempt to diffuse the violent confrontations. Jon continued to sit, whilst obviously highly agitated, and continued to listen to the cushions that preoccupied his senses. Like a manifestation of a peculiar synchronicity, all sorts of people from his past were crawling out of the woodwork, and presenting themselves to him. They were filling him with a myriad of warnings, secret information and commands. China Dolls would leap from the mantle piece and dance across the floor and they possessed a most sinister quality, their eyes haunting and penetrating. They were scaring the life out of Jon. Friends who had previously remained faithful were now upsetting him also, coming out from ebony holes with all sorts of distorted instructions and narration.

This pattern of behaviour lasted for five days and five nights. In an effort to contain the situation, the family took it in turns to keep watch over their loved one, all through the day and night. Jon would at times attack items of furniture, and race from one room to the next. His movements reached across wild trajectories, with little rational basis. His levels of energy seemed colossal, with no end to this in sight. Duke was always right behind him and he too did not sleep. He was loyal and true, his perception of Jon was still that of his master. As a consequence Duke followed him without hesitation, shadowing his every move. His affection was tangible, although Jon was not aware of it.

As Jon battered hopelessly against every opening, he felt as though he was detained without choice again. This evoked a deep and overwhelming phobia of incarceration. As his hands shook violently, Jon smoked cigarettes at a relentless pace and then they disappeared from his hands, without trace. The blankets that covered him were transformed into steel wool and felt harsh and uncomfortable. Jon was lost in deep discussion with the screaming voices in his head and in his frustration he tried in vain to break into doors in an attempt to find food, as he was also absolutely ravenous. He was overpowered by this sensory onslaught and he slumped by his entrance door, tears streaming into a well of misery. It was a time of deepest despair.

Sarah had tried to comfort him and although Jon was no longer aggressive, he did not even recognise her. She found this aspect particularly difficult and wondered where had he gone? Could a personality really become so submerged as never to return? While Sarah cradled her partner in her arms, she noticed that Jon had pulled clumps of hair from his head, leaving his scalp exposed. This seemed to be symbolic of his mental decline, of living in bleak confinement. Jon's expression was full of torment and he appeared to know no one. There would be apparitions of people from his past and present to transiently involve himself with, before they vanished, without trace. They were creating manifestations to deceive and the residue was toxic. Jon believed that his family had split into separate ego states, with a good example confronted by an evil one. Initially they seemed superficially identical, until they began to speak. Then it became apparent which side they were on. The satanic projections were horrific and laced with spirits of deception. The pure elements were initially overpowered, but Jon called up to the heavens, begging for release. As the house filled with a plethora of different characters, Jon did not know whom to trust. There were no constants and Jon found himself brimming over with rage, not knowing why. He wanted to grasp and shatter this frenzied existence and lay it to rest.

Eventually Jon came to standstill, collapsing on to his bed. He had reached the end of this crazed adventure; after the extremes of activity his body had given up. Duke lay down beside him and he was also shattered. All of those hours tending to his needs, Duke had remained faithful. Now in the aftermath Sarah and his parents had to put the house back in order. Amongst the bizarre reminders of the last few days there was money left in the frying pans, bread on the coffee tables, after shave soaked into the carpet. There was also toilet paper strewn all across the dining room and dog food on the bookcases. Jon had left behind him a trail of havoc. The family prayed that it was all over now. It had been a nightmare, both mentally and physically, and Sarah was shaking all over, still in a state of disbelief and shock. She had never experienced anything like it. Jon had adopted different personalities, none of which she was familiar with. She could not get over the fact that he did not know who she was.

Every half hour or so the family checked on Jon but he was fast asleep, as his body endeavoured to recover. He had endured an acute period of activity and they all wondered what he would be like when he awoke. Would the mania start again? It was as though he had been possessed by evil spirits, but would they now be exorcised? There were many uncertainties and questions, all of which had to be confronted and answered.

For the moment, however, the period of madness had passed.

Jon never reached that state again, but he came

close. When the manic episodes returned, the same procedure was followed, by the family locking him in the house and watching over his movements. He was propelled by a super-human energy and all they could do was to try and contain it. Predictably the lows followed as Jon sank into the most crippling depressions and was unreachable in his feelings of hopelessness. At these times he had to be nursed as though incapable of the most basic functions. Sarah fed and washed him, for he was totally dependent, all his vitality gone. Sarah suffered with him, she felt all the aching, relentless anguish. At times she wanted to withdraw and detach herself, but she could not allow this, such was her love for him. Sometimes she would go to the attic and contemplate the imagery of Jon's paintings and play his music, for they were all part of the Jon she wanted back so desperately. Sarah reflected on the poems he had written for her and the pastel studies dedicated to her, for now she was alone.

This pattern continued for several months, with Sarah adopting the role of carer. Jon's parents helped by watching over their lost son whilst Sarah rested. As time passed, Jon began to make some progress, but it was tentative. Sometimes he appeared to respond to the things he had previously created. He seemed to smile when he heard parts of the creative fusion that had been influential in his life. This was encouraging as it was a sign that things were connecting to his conscious thoughts. Sarah hoped that these elements of Jon's personality would transcend all the trials he endured. Maybe piece by piece his quality of life would be restored.

One day, out of the darkness Sarah could hear the twines of the double bass as she prepared a meal. She rushed upstairs to find Jon standing in the corner of his studio, plucking on the strings.

Overwhelmed by emotion, she ran up to him and held his withered form, squeezing him tight. She was in floods of tears, such was her feeling of relief. Sarah had yearned for this day, the time when her lover returned.

Sarah dreamed that they would be able to walk again, to talk about everything and anything, to lie under the trees and to prepare those wonderful meals. All the things that made their relationship so special. Perhaps they could go back to the Lakes, to the same cottage, with its neighbouring forests and fields. Despite all the trials and difficulties, she would never let Jon go.

Jon had alternated between the manic and the catatonic. Everything had been violently polarised, with little, if any, stability. Yet as the days passed, more of Jon's personality was revealed, all of which heralded progress. It was just painfully slow. At night as he slept, Sarah would place her hands on him and pray, earnest in her need. Jon was such a distant soul. This was evident in the mornings as he sat in the garden, smoking copious amounts of cigarettes and gazing into the distance. He was in his own little world and no one could be quite sure what was going on in his head. He was contained within an emotional cell, its interior fragmented into tiny pieces. Perhaps the only direction was to pursue a healing from the core and to believe that a miracle was possible.

Sarah was to walk forward in faith and reject any sense of doubt.

Sarah knew that Jon had always possessed a Bible and had tried to live by its teachings. The pair had prayed together and had been blessed together. Perhaps their love was a miracle in its own right as it had come from the most difficult of circumstances. They had been brought to each other by the Lord, in that they truly believed. Sarah and Jon were on the periphery of real commitment to a spiritual ideal. They were aware that this world had made Jon a broken man; how could it be expected to put him back together again? No, Jon's neurophysiological state had to be dealt with by immersion in praise and worship. Sarah offered Jon to the heavens and asked for him to be cleansed, for his spirit to be made whole again.

Sarah now had to find the right location for their worship, to be able to discover a ministry and fellowship where she and Jon would be at peace. Sarah was aware that he needed a certain prayer that penetrated the hidden parts of his mind, to plunge deeper and deeper into the past. When that point was reached, then all the pain could be bound and contained, all the experiences that had harmed could be banished.

Sarah had noticed a church in town that displayed eyecatching and emotive posters, their headlines usually taken from scripture. It was quite an imposing building, with the most stunning stained glass reflecting its glittering design across cracked and uneven pathing that framed the avenue leading from the entrance. On Sundays she had seen all sorts of people pass through its gates. The sound of praise would flow from the opened doors. She knew that this would be the place to bring themselves to.

Jon was in the living room, his face screwed up, as the voices raged and tore into his consciousness. Sarah approached him and gently held his hand. She then looked right into his eyes and smiled softly. She explained that they were to go to a church service and that he would be helped with his difficulties. To Sarah's surprise and relief Jon did not oppose the suggestion. She viewed this as Jon's last chance of healing and redemption. As days had drifted past Jon had become a little more receptive, but was still captured by the challenges of mental illness. During the nocturnal hours Sarah remembered their conversations of yesterday. She recalled the time when they professed that their lives would be together forever. For they would always be inside each other. Jon would lay down his life for Sarah, and she the same. Now they were to offer their lives to God, in their quest to find the answers to mysteries of humanity and the spiritual world, whilst tending to their emotional needs. Jon had to be nurtured back to health. Only then could they release the feelings of positivity, to walk in the hills and plunge into the sparkling waters. He could return to the park where he was as a child, talk to David and release those wretched, destructive demons. Jon had been restrained by these for most of his life, but he was still loved, still needed by those around him, which was a testament to his real worth. During those lonely passages when he seemed to have lost sight of any deliverance, he had called out to the Holy Spirit. Jon was now waiting to receive this healing, to hand over his soul in faith.

When Sunday morning arrived Sarah helped Jon to get ready. She had a strong feeling of anticipation and, more intensely, of hope. But she was not aware what form any progress would take. As they entered the church they were immediately overwhelmed by the sound of a full gospel choir. Jon proceeded to laugh and tap his foot. He intrinsically felt a warmth that penetrated deep within. Was something provoking a reaction already? The richest of harmonies were floating up to the vaulted ceiling and reverberating. The singers swayed from side to side, projecting their vocal attack and clapping their hands to the rhythm. The horn players were gesticulating towards the heavens and the pianists were bouncing on their stools. What an atmosphere! The congregation were infected by all of the joyous sounds and could only add to the sea of voices. Jon stood there, mesmerised by it all. He wanted to be part of it.

The minister then climbed up to the pulpit and the service began. There was a lot to absorb as his teachings and messages poured out in abundance. He insisted that everything that was said could be confirmed by the lessons of the Holy Word, contained in scripture. During times of prayer, individuals would speak in strange, alien tongues. This disturbed Jon somewhat until he was told by a kindly gentleman by his side that that was exactly what they were; tongues. Sometimes they were a recognised language, sometimes not. But it was an expression or gift of the spirit, and was always confirmed and translated by at least one other person. This amazed Jon and he found himself captivated by all this joyous activity around him. The preacher referred to the Old Testament initially and described the trials and torment of Job's life. Despite all of his tribulations he had pulled through the quagmire and reached an existence of even higher blessings. But it was the descriptions of the torture he endured that Jon related to the most.

For Satan had tested Job; in his attempt to turn him against God he took everything away from him. Jon knew that Job had existed with nothing, had then been given much, only to be deprived of all things of worth again. Could any of this be relevant to him? Would all his experiences be crowned by real forgiveness?

As Jon sunk into deep and truthful prayer, he was made aware that the first step forward had to come from him. For the Lord was waiting for him, to accept and to love him, despite his frailty and vulnerability. Jon dearly wanted to give back to Sarah all that she had sacrificed during the periods that she had cared for him. Gradually he found himself recognising that the internal parts of his soul that had laid dormant for years were now awakening. The preacher's words were resonating and appeared to be pertinent and applicable to his own life. From that he could not escape. The example of Job made him realise that his own life had followed a similar path.

From his seat alongside Sarah in the weathered pews, Jon turned and professed his endless love for her. In response she fell to her knees and broke down. She was enraptured, lost in Jon's affection.

It was then that a very large African man walked right through the crowd and headed straight for Jon and Sarah. It was as though the waves had been parted, such was the magnitude of his presence. He introduced himself as Shelton and explained that he was part of the Ministry team. He had noticed the pair at the back of the church, and after sensing their need had made a mental note to meet up with them after the service. He gestured for Jon and Sarah to make their way to a door to the right of the choir stalls. As they entered the room, they both felt an atmosphere of peace and tranquillity.

They sat down, on the edge of their chairs, and then Shelton began to talk. He instinctively perceived that Jon had found the teachings of Job to be most profound and in a particularly personal sense. He recognised Jon's conflict, the spiritual warfare that he had to contend with. He also realised that all of this had taken the form of mental illness. This was often the case, he explained. Frequently these battles were conveyed as a dislocation from reality, with the most extraordinary phenomena revealing themselves. But there was an answer and it was through the mysteries of faith and healing that Jon was here today.

It all seemed unerringly accurate and Jon wondered how he knew all of these things. He felt that the trivial periphery had dispersed and now the fundamental causes and patterns that had been established were to be worked upon. It would mean commitment and there would be periods where everything seemed tedious and painful. Jon was wavering somewhat and could barely hear the words Shelton was saying. As he asked Sarah to repeat them to him, she felt an incredible sense of purpose within the room. It was nothing she could tangibly get hold of, but she knew it was there. Her duty was to be Jon's backbone. He was too weak, bombarded by all manner of visions and auditory invasion.

Jon could see birds of paradise fluttering up to the open window. He called out to them, thanking them for their wondrous display of colour. Even his old friends the bricks were making their presence felt. He could not judge whether this was to be a good omen or otherwise, whether they were portending a blessing or curse. Shelton took hold of his hand, and spoke of prophetic signification. These images were to tell the story of Jon's inner world. They should not be ignored or trivialised, as had happened in the past at the institutions. There was much they could reveal. But first, it was time to say a prayer. Opening Jon's mind and soul to the power of God was the first step.

Jon and Sarah continued to go to the church, although at times Jon would have to leave the service because he felt he was burning in the heat of spiritual elements in confrontation. But as he sat outside, he would listen to the power of the vocal praise, which still reached him from a distance.

The pace of the healing was leaden, but now Jon was able to pick up his pen and write, expressing his emotions. He would also sit at the piano keyboard, as he had done when first familiarising himself with chords. He had also painted the purest rose, in full bloom and in tender coral, leaving it for Sarah. When she walked into the bedroom and saw it, she was so moved that words all but eluded her.

Shelton visited every week, at times more frequently when the need arose, as Jon was still unstable. Shelton was full of patience and was a man of great learning. He made references to scripture that were consistently accurate. To Jon he had become his teacher and his doctrine was enlightening.

During times of prayer Jon would sometimes holler and shout expletives, demonstrating all manner of demonic projections. But Shelton seemed prepared for this and would reassure Sarah that it was all part of the healing process. It appeared that the closer Jon got to the truth, the greater the interference. He would writhe on the carpet, barking like a wounded hound. Sarah allowed herself to be led by Shelton and focus her spiritual intuition. That was her strength, which she used to help overcome this hellish onslaught.

Jon's periods in the studio were becoming more fruitful, however. Concurrently he was evolving his own visual language, but in a new context. He would labour at the easel, manipulating the mediums to create bold new images. The first time Shelton was allowed to see his work, he was impressed. He could not believe that this was all produced by one man. Its scope and breadth was extensive, a staggering projection of talent. As Shelton attempted to absorb the enormity of it all, he realised that here an inroad could be made into Jon's troubled mind and unravelling the semantics of his written and spoken words could reveal much, as Jon was so misaligned and confused.

It was like entering a maze for the first time.

In the mornings, as Jon drank his coffee and smoked the first cigarette, he would comment that it was a funny old world. Sarah had heard him say it a hundred times, and knew that it was not a flippant remark. It really was that strange to him.

She too regarded Shelton as the wise man. But they needed to contact their angel, for they yearned for protection from pain. One day Jon would take Sarah back to the cedar tree again, to a time when their anguish had first evaporated.

It began with rain, torrents of it. Streams of the skies' water were challenging the efficiency of mankind's decrepit drainage systems. But unbeknown to Jon and Sarah this day would develop into something monumental. Jon was resting in the studio, a paint brush still in his hand. Sarah came up and looked at him for a while, not knowing for how long. His expression was peaceful, his brow for once relaxed. As she concentrated on his face, she noticed that underneath the lids, his eyes were flickering, lost in the realms of R.E.M. She picked up a piece of note paper from his desk and tried to read it, but it was unintelligible, just a haphazard pattern of scrawls. She wondered what had been going through his mind at the time. It seemed as though he was beginning to stir, and she wanted to be with him when he did. There was an apparent aura about him and she did not want to lose this special quality. She wanted to let him wake.

But the moment passed, as he remained lost in his deep sleep. She looked up through the skylight: the rain was still drumming, but the sun was shining through and the spectrum lit the firmament. The beauty of the rays only illuminated her feelings of relative insignificance. Some specks of oil paint had hit the floorboards and Sarah stared at them, following the grain. She began to ruminate, whilst contemplating the most demanding dimension of living with the madness, especially the occasions when Jon did not recognise her any more.

Sarah recalled the times when she and Jon could not stop whooping and cheering, the periods when they were immersed in frivolity and fun. For Jon's basic character was coloured by an incisive wit, but he was more like a dependent baby now. She could just sit, watch and think about him. Sarah had been reassured by the congregation of their church that a lot of prayer had been dedicated to them both. Meanwhile, Jon's parents could not always cope with seeing him and to be honest, Sarah understood. They still regarded him as their child, a vulnerable youth to protect and to nurture. This approach was inappropriate, of course, but that was how they dealt with their only son. There were times when they could stand no more and it was then that they walked away.

Sarah decided to make a pot of Earl Grey and to keep it warm for when Jon opened his eyes. She sensed that it would not be too long, as there were ripples of consciousness apparent from his relaxed muscles. In the corner of the room was Jon's African drum and Sarah picked it up, caressing the skin and then proceeding to tap out a gentle rhythm. Before long Sarah felt quite dreamy and felt her own eyelids becoming heavier. But she resisted the feeling, just holding onto the sense of relaxation.

Jon then mumbled something incomprehensible and awoke with a start. He was initially disorientated, but Sarah was there before him and he smiled, as her face was familiar. They then took tea, but for a while did not speak, as there was no need, for all communication was through their body language. Jon reached forward and grasped Sarah's hand, as he had had the most vivid of dreams.

He had been on the edge of a desert, which was defined by the most hostile of terrains and he had nothing to protect himself with, being naked and exposed. Before his eyes was a scorpion, its tail curled, ready to attack. He could envisage the poison running into his veins, and then the creature grew into a monster. It retained the same form, but had escalated in scale. Jon realised that there was no escape and that he had reached the end of his life on this earth. It was then that he called to the heavens, crying out for life beyond this worldly despair and to be released from his sins. There was then an almighty explosion, resulting in a luminous glow and all conflict was released. Jon thought that he had screamed out loud, but Sarah had not heard a thing. He was not full of the fear when he woke that he had expected, for he had been given the most conclusive reassurance. There had been a projection of light all around, with an intensity that he could not deny. This illumination signified the transformation of energy from darkness to light, reaching the heart of Jon's soul and leaving him with the release of true redemption. He had now left the convoluted path that was leading him to perpetual torment.

Jon and Sarah sat and talked about this experience for what had seemed like hours. There had been a spiritual linkage to their own relationship and the bond was solidifying. Jon became animated in a way that had eluded him for an age. As he picked up drawings, they now made sense and a lot of his literary ramblings were brought into coherent shape.

Sarah did not want to discuss themes of insanity, those reflections provoked by the extremes of Jon's precarious mental health. She preferred to concentrate on her role in Jon's life in the present tense. She believed that their companionship was to adapt, leading to greater fulfilment and hopefully stability. Jon did not want to regress, or to be taken back to care in an institution. He decided go to see his parents soon and of his own volition. He would tell them of his love and respect, telling them to worry no more. In response they were to keep providing support and be forgiving, despite their periods of consternation.

There was more to evolve between these haunted individuals, maybe resulting in a catalyst of emotion that would resolve and tend to those wounds that remained open and gaping. As Sarah and Jon prayed in earnest, they were both provided with images that illustrated the love that flowed between them, like an entwining cord. The pair could see their flesh bonded together and there was now a real feeling of expectancy as they faced each and every day.

As the pair continued to pray, it became clear that they must not leave the studio. For what reason it had not yet transpired. They were to lie on the floor, side by side. The patter of rain-fall had ceased and a white light emanated from the roof opening. Sarah was guided by an impulse to lay her hand upon Jon's temples. She reached them with her finger tips that were outstretched to their limit. Jon felt the most incredible warmth, which passed through his whole body as though it was being covered with warm honey. He recalled that Shelton had informed them that this often happened when the Spirit was called and then absorbed. It was not long before Sarah experienced the same sensation, but from the edge of her legs which were pressed against Jon's. It too filled her, to the point of brimming over. There was also the apparent sound of music in the background, transmitted by the strains of a cathedral organ. Then the sound of bells, ringing in unison, filled the room like an auditorium as though it were a Church.

They were called to kneel by the commands that they heard and although the flooring was hard, they were not uncomfortable. They held their hands together and waited, wondering what would be laid before them. They remained in silence, until there was a roar, seemingly emanating from the walls. They jumped back in fright, before the sound of tongues transformed into the ethereal tone of the voices of angels, which took the form of humans and appeared from the brickwork, blessing Jon and Sarah. The eyes of these angelic beings possessed a silver sheen, their skin the whitest of white. They radiated goodness, being the personification of purity and innocence. They floated above Sarah and Jon, pouring Holy water upon them and then vanished into a void. There was a rush of warm air and it was all over. Jon turned to look at Sarah and she smiled, her face full of brightness and calm. Everything now seemed complete. The Lord had arrived, they had seen Him and He had spoken to this loving pair. The four walls of their house now felt secure. The angels had brought absolute assurance and now opened the path for Jon and Sarah to step forward in faith. They would never perceive the world in the same way. There would no doubt and no helplessness for the demons had been banished, their hold on this segment of humanity broken. No one had known of the timing, but God Himself. But now there was to be no denial, nor conflict, for the torrents that raged into the darkest hours had eased and there was to be no more of the beast of disorder. Jon and Sarah held each other and gave thanks.

Now the healing was overflowing and they could see, further than ever before.

CHAPTER FIVE – GLORY

Despite the fullness of the experience of redemption, there were times when Jon felt alone, deep in the quest to further his sense of wellbeing. There remained sounds in his head, but these took the form of a humming, as though a reverberation of beauty. This enabled him to reach the crests and to survive the descent into the troughs. Jon spent many an hour observing the stretching of the skin protecting life below the water level of ponds and lakes; the dragonflies resting on the film, as all the subtleties and nuances of nature revealed themselves. That was part of the fascination, as Jon imagined what micro-organisms existed beneath the surface. He was immersing himself in themes of relativity and the beauty of this earth.

Within his subconscious Jon fleetingly located himself within the autumnal tones of the forest. It was approaching night-time, but Jon was not fearful as the sounds of nature provided him with the spiritual sustenance to combat any concerns. As Jon observed the linear growth of the pine trees, he was aware that he was in pursuit of elegant, natural forms. When he diverted his attention to the contrasting memory of the school-yard, where he had fallen victim to the most sadistic cruelty, he was transported to the heaving metropolis, where he was just another faceless figure, lost in the intoxication of the hustle and bustle. Jon was being carried from dream reality to heightened reality.

LIVES WITHIN A LIFE

The studio had been elevated in terms of its emotional value and was providing a retreat for Jon and Sarah. The reality of the angels penetrating the depths of their being was still vivid and the influence of God's teachings was huge. As they focused beyond the outlet from the skylight above, seasons came and went, as did the patterns of their spirits and moods. The verse that Jon had created was becoming all the more prophetic, with rapid holy confirmation of its content as they immersed themselves in what was becoming the greatest venture of all. The pair were pushing back the boundaries from this base, with Jon aware that when he stroked the plaster of the walls as he passed by; it was an indication of his feelings of security, for Sarah and he had found their sanctuary.

Jon dreamed of floating on the ascending swirl, of flying like an aeroplane above the clouds. In the past there were occasions when Jon would assimilate mental impressions from a detached vantage point.

Looking down he saw instances of mutilation and torture, which could be related to his own life. He wished these could be replaced with joy, to be able to pursue happiness as a gift.

Jon and Sarah considered that their past was comparable to existing on the wilder trajectories of turbulent travel and encountering unexplained phenomena. They wanted their creations to grow to wider proportions and bring the ethos of collective compassion to fruition. For now their scars had paled.

Along the road, they found examples of creation that were ultimately rejected. All facets of imagery, literature and sound were appraised frequently as the complexities of their meaning were unravelled. Often all manner of polarised and unintelligible semantics were uncovered and that was why the structure was so crucial. Jon and Sarah assembled all parts in painstaking detail since the delivery had to be flawless.

Jon and Sarah were calling out to the destitute who line the walkways and alleyways of the city. They were the forlorn, with no pleasure to grasp, no chances, or choices. Their existence was dictated by a relentless loneliness and persecutory despair. But were they really living beyond the trials of insanity, existing in a world that could never be appreciated or understood?

Jon had been a boy with fear in his eyes, but no one even noticed. He was full of words that nobody read or attempted to decipher. Instead he had found his companionship with the stability of bricks and mortar and the contrasting birds of flight. They were the only entities that provided any consistency in his desperate existence. But now he was to stand above it all, for he had been called by God.

LIVES WITHIN A LIFE

Jon was emerging from a war zone, where the protagonists had been laid to rest. Strategies were evolving and were to be revealed through his master plan. Across the deserted patches of Jon's mind lay memories of the injured and the deceased. In the process of exorcising demons there had been much destruction. Humanity's genetic material had been passed down from generation to generation, in the form of fragmented pieces. That battle ground was part of an enormous puzzle; facets of a man, revealing the darker side, from behind the face presented to the world. Jon considered his own development to have mutated at the point of his conception. This notion had occurred to both Jon and Sarah and they felt that their eyes had been opened. It was both fascinating and gruesome, but a real discovery.

Shelton would be present with them at times, sometimes apparent in voice only, drifting through their consciousness. An image of David, which Jon had clung to for all those years, would become alive and vibrant and was full of praise for their attempts to realise dreams. He was a man who had lived a rich and abundant life, despite losing his sanity. But his presence remained immediate; Jon would never erase his memories of David, which remained fond.

Jon's parents were still together after all those years but were now withered and grey. But they were consistently loving for they regarded Jon as precious. They always returned to their son, embracing him with warmth and were there during times of need, even when they themselves were lost.

The systems that control reasoning had eluded Jon for prolonged periods. But now he was being propelled to pastures new, with an uprising of the soul. He felt like a rocket surging to the core of creative activity, deflecting all intrusion, transforming his thoughts from barbaric bombardment to passionate escapism. All destructive links in his ancestry were now laid to rest.

Jon and Sarah had visited the most uninhabitable places of the human condition on their voyage. They had endured the endless nights and the harshness of the impact when plunging to the depths of emotional ravines. But wherever they were taken, the two were connected, with their thoughts being transmitted, one to the other. Their feelings of acute vulnerability had now dissipated. They climbed trees, releasing the child inside them and swung from the branches, avoiding the pollution of this earth. However, beyond the stillness there was the sound of thunder in the distance. Like the skies struggling to contain the weight of moisture and resonance of dynamic activity, it felt as though it was coming ever closer.

Jon and Sarah were aware that they had to be careful when facing disturbing experiences, as many people had become deranged beyond recognition whilst submerged in realities from the past. But as they surfed over the summits and into introspective caverns, their feelings of empowerment and their stamina were maintained. Together they would silence any threat, as their sense of direction was strengthened.

Jon and Sarah felt compelled to put together their own ministry, with the substance of their trials to be conveyed with conviction. They continued to draw from their own discoveries and to put them into context. When they prayed in earnest, the pair were provided with an image of a dome, a place where the fusion of visionary healing would take place. It was to be the most colossal outpouring of emotion. Those who were broken by life would come in their droves, for they understood how despair could destroy their intrinsic spirit. The wounds and gashes that represented years of mutilation were to be banished, like a flare that lights up the course of humanity.

Jon and Sarah were thrust into the mesmerising flow of a dominant convergence, appearing out of nowhere. It seemed to be all part of God's mysterious power and it was bewitching. When they surfaced from the crash of the waves, they would testify the content of their enlightened minds and witness to the crowds of lost souls. Their volumes of acquired knowledge were to be shared, to nurture those in need.

Jon and Sarah were projected into a room made up of numerous unbalanced angularities. There was no cohesion of line, as everything suggested a heavy ugliness that was unsatisfactory to the eye. Their gaze was directed downwards, evoking a negative ambience that was overpowering. The flooring was streaked with marks that resembled a map of arteries visible through the flesh. The room was sparsely furnished and there were no windows to provide a break from the relentless, bland tones. There was no fire or passion evident in this place of sober restraint, only an air of antiseptic cleanliness that permeated all. The walls were bright white and were bare and unadorned. They were crying out for colour, for a vivid splash of luminous pigment to liven up the senses. Jon and Sarah felt that they had been taken to a place that possessed no soul. A place where there was no life to speak of, where all feeling had been stripped away. It was devoid of any positive intensity and as a consequence evoked feelings of sadness and loneliness.

They sat in the only two chairs and listened to a roar of white noise. There was nothing but a void that sucked them inwards. They were lost in a chasm, a gulf where there was nothing to stimulate, nothing to evoke excitement. When they tried to speak, no words came out. When they tried to move, they could not. The pair were losing control and the atmosphere had started to become increasingly frightening as Jon and Sarah could not communicate; even their facial muscles were frozen. They had walked into a nightmare and it seemed that they could not leave. They had become prisoners in a cell where all signs of humanity had been taken away. There were no points of reference, no areas that resembled normality.

The couple had plunged into a place where vociferous exclamation did not register, as there was no one else to sense their desperation. Inside they were battling with a joint compulsion to channel this confinement of their mind, body and soul in an attempt to control their own pained perception of an empty environment. They could only compare this enforced situation to being held, face down, on the floor of a seclusion room: a dungeon where any rights were stripped away and thrown to the beasts at the door. The blandness that was evident here, however, was all encompassing and as a consequence, provided no flame to do battle with. For there was nothing to relate to in terms of emotive predisposition or instinctive reaction. Everything seemed to have been drained away, with nothing remaining that could offer hope.

But Jon and Sarah still had their thoughts and these were the key to solving this frustrating puzzle. For despite the conditions they had found themselves in, their minds were still free. So they surmised that liberty was to be found through their intrinsic spiritual make-up, qualities that were emphatic and undeniable. The only solution, they decided, was to pray and they joined together in an attempt to overcome the isolation.

There was no response, at least for what seemed a long while. The emptiness was still dominant, reaching the nucleus of their being. But they persisted and then listened for any answer.

They had been given their own minds and so, with it, choice. The concept of free will was a complex issue to Jon and Sarah, for in their past they had survived the flame of suicidal pain and had had to reconcile these demands to the teachings of biblical text. However, from that point they had decided to step forward in faith. They needed to trust, to profess their adherence to a philosophy of giving. As they continued to pray, time was taken out of context, seeming to stretch and contort, as the void encompassed their perception of existence, leaving Jon and Sarah with nothing to apply relativity to. The brightness was overwhelming, burning their eyes, tearing into the receptors of the mind. This experience was a test, a battle between the secular world and the yearning for heavenly acceptance. The pair persisted until they could give no more, the passage pushing them further downwards, spiralling into the bowels of hell. They endeavoured to articulate their desperation, but could not be heard. The key to their imprisonment seemed to have been thrown into a raging, effervescent river.

It was at that moment that they were transported through space and taken from the room of emptiness and they then found themselves, side by side, in the studio, where everything that revealed Jon's idiosyncrasies was created. The difference was emphatic, for the walls were splattered with rich spectrums of colour and the flooring was a sea of dots, similar to the canvas of an inspired impressionist. Through the window opening the beams of the radiant sun illuminated everything before them. Harmonious diminished chords could be heard from the speaker cones positioned in the corner. Sheets of paper were strewn across the drawing desks and boards carried the multiple layers of oil paint. Shadows were cast but possessed no ominous tone for they provided a sense of visual lucidity, carving out a clarity wherever they were witnessed. Sensations of ardour, glow and vivacity were all apparent. These represented the shades and defining foundations that make up life and had affected Jon and Sarah. As conveyed by the messages of religious doctrine, they were aware that timing cannot be predicted but an eventual answer can be assured. Their joint commitment and dedication had provided the escape from an aching hollow, for now passion was all embracing. The contrast was immense and undeniable, as though etched in exquisitely patterned marble. The spread of effulgent light was now omnipresent.

From onerous sorrow Jon and Sarah had grown stronger, for their sense of purpose and belief was galvanised. But they considered the plight of those lost individuals, who were imprisoned in that room for a lifetime. Where could they find solace? Would they know the way out and be able to recognise the escape route? In response, Jon was thrown into turmoil. He felt for those who shared the melancholy, the nightmare that shattered lives. A collective body had to be formed to enable the release of compassion and expand, replacing the voices, visions and confusion.

Within their retreat Jon and Sarah had been propelled forwards by their emotional passage.

But they were not weary, for there was a profusion of stimuli to propel them ever forwards.

Periods of deliberation were required, in order to attain true clarity, as the motion of everyday life was left in trust, gently ticking away. As their minds had been cast back to the years of terror, the progression in Jon and Sarah's lives was quite remarkable. They had followed their dreams and made them tangible, living them out despite the brutality of this world.

Now the fusion of all benevolent elements was nearing completion. From their extensive travels Jon and Sarah had returned to their home. They had reached the end of the first passage of their expedition and had collected a variety of different sights, words, and sounds. Now it was time to collate and combine them all whilst conveying the beauty of their relationship with each other and the art of juxtaposing relevant imagery. Most importantly, the fundamental aspects of their destiny were now collected. The final part of the preparation was now ready to begin.

The dreamscapes contained within their imagination were to fuel the eventual proceedings. For the immediate future, however, Jon and Sarah were to sit back and to prepare themselves through meditation and internal focus.

The components serving their philanthropic

outlook were: imagery, verse and sound. They had all been assembled with invariable accuracy in order to create something greater than the sum of their parts. The transportation to different lands and experiences of life was to provide the foundation. Then the intricacies of detail were applied, layer upon layer, as though constructing an immense skyscraper. There were facets of subconscious experience to be incorporated, arranged into a system, revealing reflections and prominent memories that pierced the surface. These formed a basis for the presentation of projected imagery, beginning with initial studies of anatomy, then progressing through expressionism, to cubism, abstraction and conceptualism. Much of this was sourced from Jon's own visual experimentation and it formed a distinct pattern. Placed upon this were the verse and literature that were sourced from years of recording aspects of life through a multitude of journals. They would be arranged chronologically, with references ranging from the Biblical to the philosophical. Finally there would be the collages of sound, containing rhythmic structures, timbre, cadence, and then the cathedral, from where the acoustics would float to the heavens and all elements would peak. This would lead to the finality, built upon all of the other parts. The location for the ultimate projection would be a golden dome above the earth, looking down from space.

The whole vision would be concurrently seen, felt and heard until a catalyst formed and only then would the reawakening be complete.

This was to be the final journey, an accumulation of years of trial and tribulation. But these years had been fused together, creating a wall of intense invigoration. Jon and Sarah had developed a capacity to bear vast loads, their minds capable of extreme mental gymnastics. Now it was time to apply their knowledge.

Jon and Sarah lay down, holding each other with tenderness and sensitivity. They felt enticed by a persuasive force to look up to the ceiling and their eyes moved together as though synchronised. The beams that framed the ceiling were taken apart, moving to the edges of the walls and a huge screen appeared. It took over the whole of the vault, but all that could be seen was an intense illumination that spread over a vast area. There was no form, just a luminous glow. The pair were spellbound, not even daring to blink. Then the deepest of blues framed the ensuing spectacle. It was as though they were to be submerged in the wash of the sea's awesome power. All of this stimulus was intoxicating, leading Jon and Sarah into a separate reality that was warm and welcoming. They considered that their cerebral powers were reaching new and previously unattainable heights. The pair were riding on a missile of intellectual and sensory projection.

Then there was a distant rumble, gradually gaining in might, like a storm moving ever closer. The supporting walls seemed to quiver and shake in response. Ripples of motion from the oak flooring travelled right through the bodies of the chosen couple. The experiences that had shaped them led up to their final, joint purpose and was all displayed before their alert eyes, flashing past them: the initial innocence that had been transformed into the onset of derangement, accompanied by abuse and imprisonment; the wealth of creativity, inspired by loss and grief, together with the seemingly endless periods of isolation and confusion; the times of self-harm, highlighted by the spiritual warfare. But eventually the relief of reciprocal love and adoration between Jon and Sarah was triumphant. All of this was shown as it had occurred, their existence from conception until the present. All paths had led to this and now there was no sense of denial for the picture was complete as Jon and Sarah had been given absolute truth, with no more to question.

The next step was the immersion in the Holy water, in order to be truly cleansed. As Jon and Sarah looked into the pool, it glistened invitingly, yet they were aware that they must wait and contain their impatience. They stood, facing one another, with their arms outstretched and their palms held upwards. It was then that the convergence of energy flooded through them both. They began to tremble, as it reached their every fibre. They were to be washed, with all impurities flushed away. The darker aspects of their souls and minds were to be no more. They were then instructed to bow down and pour the water across their foreheads. It trickled along to their open mouths and the taste was sweet.

They knelt down on mats coloured in blood red and gave thanks. As their backs arched, they felt the sensation of skin touching skin. There was a closeness apparent that surpassed everything. The Holy water was now reduced to spots of fluid, shining in the candle light. But the cleansing experience would live on forever. It was a monumental advance into an existence that was of complete peace and redemption. For now they were moving ever closer to the point when the power of faith would transcend all. They were to sit, maintaining a soothing silence for many hours, only aware of each other and God, who was radiating over them.

Jon and Sarah used this time to focus their thoughts and to remove anything that would be an obstacle or a potential threat to the equilibrium they sought after. When they opened their eyes, all they could see was a dome, resplendent in glory. It would not be long now before everything materialised as God intended. Those abstracted from normality would find their home and their deprivation would be over. Their endless days and nights spent wandering through dimly lit streets, begging for sustenance and for a cessation to the misery of an empty life existing on the periphery of society. As the privileged walked by, they did not care or want to see what was beneath their feet - the cry and call of those desperate for companionship, articulating their need for someone to reach out to them with benevolence and to break the cycle of despair.

LIVES WITHIN A LIFE

The day had come. Jon and Sarah reacted to the anticipation stirring their senses as their hands trembled and their rate of breathing accelerated. In preparation they ate simply and bathed in the coolest of water, bringing about feelings of freshness and alertness. Through the opening in the roof was a variegation of light, like a rainbow, with one colour bleeding into the next. The overall atmosphere was a combination of peacefulness and expectancy, with nothing to threaten or disturb it. A breeze passed by, snaking through this special place. Then the sound of a stream rushed past and the wind through a sea of firs, accentuating their contented mood. Exotic species of birds from the past could be seen, their vivid colouring contrasting with the deep green foliage. On the horizon the tones were all blending into one. In the centre was the cedar. It had always been there and would remain. The institutions were now ghost towns, still harbouring demons, but soon they would all be swept away.

All the parts of the spiritual embodiment that Jon and Sarah had weaved together were to be offered upwards, reverberating in their praise of humanity and tenderness. Their release and their enormity would be absorbed by all.

It was now time to travel. Jon and Sarah were to be transported to the foot of the dome. It was positioned above the earth's atmosphere and could be seen by all in its entirety. Mankind was brought together as one body and was able to reach the dome's summit by its own powers, but it was not an arduous task. No part of this was a trial, as all adversity had come before. The passage through time and space was immediate and the people were brought to this place as had been promised to them. The degree of precision was palpable, and now the release of complete healing was imminent. The dome was radiating with a brilliance and was ready to release its wonder upon the world.

The sky filled with silver rain, but no one could feel the pulse of its droplets. They were simply absorbed with no strain or tension. There were four rainbows visible, each superimposed upon the next. Their spectrum of expressive colouring was poignant. The cloud formations above provided a striking shield from the sun and were imbued with the most intense shade of aquamarine. Columns of precious metals reflected gloss and sheen whilst gleaming as the air was pure and still. Jon and Sarah stood by the peak, silently, their bodies entwined. This was the climax of a lifetime of struggle. All the materials of this union had been transformed into persuasive spiritual matter. The dome was preserving this in its wonder now as all periods of friendless scattering had passed over. Nothing more could be done to attain true freedom. Now all that was left was the timing of the launch and the release of triumph and glory.

LIVES WITHIN A LIFE

Out of nowhere came a crescendo of strings and woodwind, followed by a choral adagio that poured over the senses like a bath of luxuriant juices. From this an immense rhythmic fortress was to emerge that held all the melodic experimentation in place. Its roots were secure and dependable, locking together the layers of wild flurries that explored desires and affection. Synthesised sound pads captured each phrase with confidence and grandeur. Invisible virtuosos were leading this extensive work and its attempts to define the beauty of mankind's condition. This all led into a cataclysmic symphony, within which the symbolism and imagery were profound. Angels came down from the heavens and vocalised in unison. There were explorations into areas of improvisation, held together with the counterpoints and choruses of the now contented masses. The memories of darker times were played in minor keys, with a more strident and awkward accent. Placed in the centre of the mix was the twine of deepest frequencies, a bass swell which all on earth could hear. As the reverberation caused the ground to quake, the layers of bowed strings felt like cashmere on chilled skin. The placing of sparse, modal chords penetrated deep within, a place where a movement of emotion released both tears and the most affecting trials of existence. Sequences of seemingly random notation were generating a tidal wave of intense, challenging impressions. So here was the auditory diary that Jon and Sarah had compiled, its content both inspiring and disturbing. All those facets of the human subconscious were contained within improvised excursions into acoustic expression. Jon recalled the occasions when he could hear music emerging from the crests and waves of the ocean, as patterns of sound formed a linkage in his forever searching brain. The steady hum of passing traffic that never seemed to end became the basis of a meditative tone that was capable of soothing the troubled mind. Those crazy birds of the woods called and chatted with a vivacity and sense of playful animation. They inspired areas of Jon's creative zones to inject elements of frivolity and provide a balance to the depths of his memories of mental despair. Even the abstracted rustle of fallen leaves in the autumnal wind provoked alternative senses of artistic direction. When Jon and Sarah were lost in intense communication, he felt a compulsion to capture the essence of all of these sources of emphatic stimulation. The influence of the most valued recordings in Jon's collection had all contributed to this acoustic alchemy. From the initial crackle on the turntable, when needle makes contact with vinyl, to the close of a vibrant symphony, the passage was full of turns and twists that all culminated in serenity and peace.

Then there was the sonority of a melodious chorus, followed by a common gasp as all the sounds became one, and they rose to the towers that framed the aperture. The root of every chord was incisive and contributed to a vast and inspired musical landscape. The cathedral that symbolised the receptacle to the dome then opened its doors to the imagery and verse. The music had begun and would conclude the whole journey.

LIVES WITHIN A LIFE

Canvases projecting the most evocative of images were displayed as though on vast pieces of celluloid stretched over a substantial frame. Light passed through them and ignited their content with lucidity and tenderness. They formed a semi circle, rather like a dome of smaller proportions captured within a larger dome. Aspects of oppression that influenced perception as though casting shadows were reshaped into an emotional depth that would transcend the fervent nature of mental challenge. Just as there were flaws in the surface of canvas material, these could be converted into representations of the complexities of this earth. Art and all manifestations of creative output were here to offer a sense of order to history and worldly and spiritual events. Culture, in all its aspects, reflected the ultimate passage or journey. Lining the periphery of the proceedings were sculptures cast in bronze, carved from marble, or made of composites. They were arranged against the walls with the tallest first, so as to create a convincing force and power. They formed their own illusion of space that all could relate to. Just to convey the wonder of the human anatomy was to display a miracle of nature. There was also evident within the posture of these carved marble bodies the resilience and vulnerability of us all. Tears of sadness would run down the furrowed cheeks like discarded candle wax. These rivers of emotion etched and made their mark on every face, in every land. This shared notion brought people together, bringing about concepts of unity and relativity. The instances where internal imagery could be universally related to shone with blinding clarity. So the towering form of the human physique and its athleticism stood above, prompting feelings of wonderment.

From the intensity of urban nightmares to meanderings along the contours of battered coastlines, the propensity of man to experience fear was confronted and left to dissipate into the cloud formations above. Within the collective mind a command of light was directed into inner recesses and so dispensed with the terror of psychological incarceration. Inspiration that had been derived from those studies of nature had taken away any harshness or burning sensation that signalled raw emotion. The serenity of impressionistic strokes and the fire of expressionistic sweeps heralded a vivacity which could empower and distract the mind from any intrusion. Those combined marks and layers only went to take the eye to the summit where all would be revealed. From that vantage point false icons of the age were exposed for their true worth, as there was little to redeem them.

The eruption of this creative trinity was tantalisingly close to the troubled masses, for the projection of heavenly authority was imminent.

The gentlest of hues made their presence felt upon Jon and Sarah, manifested by a sensation of animated and swirling under-currents that enveloped the body. Just as visual symbols could penetrate and inspire, so too the neurophysiology of their brain matter was responding with resounding buoyancy. From these evocations, the caress of a brush captured and reflected radiant light from behind hidden enclosures. Places where casualties lay on the lawns of the asylum, staring at the sky, deprived of love and affection. They were the tormented, those who could only relate to extremes of isolation. But when the compositions stood, visible to the earth, so those abstracted were flooded with light. They were bathing in the rays emitted by an emotional beacon. There were times when those individuals would cower in the profusion of corridors leading to a myriad of back wards, stripping them of their humanity. The screams were heard in the darkest of nights, as torn nails scraped down the borders of the cells of confinement. But in the present, their eyes were faced with kaleidoscopic impressions of chromatic colouring as bugs and insects tested the strength of the membrane protecting organisms beneath the lake's surface. Those lost souls were being led to a place of sanctuary and all-encompassing safety. The passing of seemingly endless years had now eased their pain, covering over those flame-red scars and lacerations. The assimilation of graphically realised truths was to be a crucial element in this vast, far-reaching transformation. The healing would impress upon the heart and relieve it of its burden.

Jon and Sarah felt they were communicating with those in need and also with those who remained in a state of resistance and did not want to hear. There were those who felt unable to accept an alternative approach to life. Yet the pair truly believed that anything was possible. They wanted to allow an emotional blending of their benevolent ethos and a broad palette of experience to augment the flow and momentum of releasing demons. The bricks that were formed from the subtle qualities of limestone provided a source and root for a transcending journey to the heavens. This was a place where the most extreme and eclectic collection of individuals could find deliverance and where angels displayed their ethereal virtues by way of balletic animation. This expression of evocative movement could be made permanent by the use of economical marks and etching, as the tonality of line and form was ready to be recorded. At the other end of the spectrum, a fierce savagery was conveyed by a deliberate visual invocation to remove unclean spirits. This allowed the flow of textural patterns and the absorption of those wild and beautiful colours that offered a poetic freedom. They responded to the demands of this flawed and distorted world. Jon and Sarah were to be led into a fabulous entrance to the penultimate place of worship, the cathedral, where every perfectly formed element would pour over the sick and oppressed in a manner akin to the torrent of a warm, sensuous waterfall. It would lead the sick to the dome. Lining the periphery, were figures held in faultless repose, for they had been frozen in a state of absolute tranquillity, a place where equilibrium had been discovered. Elaborately decorated vaults spanned the vista above, seeming to stretch into infinity. They provided a guide to entice the senses through the cloudless skyscape and into the resting place of heavenly angels. From their vantage point, every permutation of the human state could be witnessed. If any particle of degradation was apparent, it would be cleansed and banished. Jon and Sarah were being used by these forces to lead the healing of a planet that was losing any remaining fragments of challenge. For now the multitude were close to a miraculous conclusion.

It was now the turn of literature, the stuff of language. Jon recalled times of crawling on his hands and knees, offering his soul to the Lord, in utter desperation. He endeavoured to articulate those acute feelings, to convey the enormity of it all. Jon had longed to throw himself from the highest summit and into the raging streams below. Whilst converting these experiences into prose, he was achieving a much desired cathartic release. This could be transposed into a language that all could relate to and share; those marks of royal blue ink soaking into the paper, only to be duplicated as a record of moments in time. Pages were turning as though they were animated, with a will of their own. These descriptions were captivating, drawing the observer forever inwards.

The collection of these accrued passages conveyed the content of years spent howling at the opaque night skies, tearing into the darkly spiritualised self. There was now a pertinence that was indisputable. The necessity was to interpret the fragility and potential of humanity and clarify those essential factors. There were now words spreading over page after page.

Jon recalled sitting on the steps of a ghetto neighbourhood, absorbing the pulse of the city as the world revolved around him. There was the steady drone of the passing traffic as the immediate atmosphere was contaminated by the stench of relentless pollution. Neon signs illuminated vast towers that appeared to grow into the heavens. The metropolis harboured a thousand faces that no one even noticed. Beneath the pavements were the sewers that bred the rodents and the sub-cultures that still survived for unfathomable reasons. The sociological complexities involved were immense and deeply affecting.

The letters that illuminated the pages describing this intricate maze seemed to be miles tall, their message spreading across the oceans, the mass of continents. Although Jon found this quite extraordinary, he was not surprised.

All he could do was to assimilate every phrase and to listen to the ebb and flow of a man of prose fulfilling his purpose. Spontaneity was balanced by reflective pathos.

Jon had managed to capture within his hardened palms facets of subconscious experience and shape them into a narrative. This appealed to and inspired those victims yearning to destroy the hold of an enforced seclusion that they had never escaped from. He had utilised the teachings of the wise men of philosophy and religion and allowed the angels to recite verses of scripture, piece by piece, whilst reinforcing principal elements when the need arose. When a broken man fell to the dusty floor, Jon related this to his own upbringing, for there were times when only a grunt was heard when he offered a prayer. Over the generations there had been individuals who had captured the quintessence of nature and man's relationship to it. Jon had previously spent many an hour confronted by ferocious waves by the sea front and the dense vegetation of forests, as they covered the mass beneath. These particles of reflection were only adding to the truth of Jon and Sarah's outpouring, their desire to connect. So, their role was not only to lead but also to provide compassion and take those in need to a spiritual asylum where oppression no longer existed. Jon now sat, remembering those whose hearts had been broken, their voices cracked and weak, as the hounds cried out from the endless backstreets, calling for the fragmented and shattered. Yet, as instinct dictated, they were still trying to pick up all the pieces, even if some particles would never be found. They were lost in the deepest caverns, somewhere far from the surface.

Now arms of angelic beings were outstretched, ready and willing to embrace the frailty of the human condition and divert all demonic influence to the dungeons of this earth. All evil and malediction was stripped of its sustenance, leaving it to wither and die, like a plant in the months of drought. For those affected, their monsters were to be confined into all of the tomorrows, their domination no more.

The writings shaped by this sublime power were now accessible to all for the book would never be closed. Soon, every lost part would be saved and crowned. The transformation would become a constant in a disturbed world.

The harmonic layers of sound that were suspended in readiness were beginning to penetrate. As the transference of energy occurred, a path conducted all of the assembled imagery and literature, which acted as roots and a foundation. They were present so as to allow the symphonies to soar into heavenly spheres. There would be that achingly beautiful quality that permeated the soul, whilst uplifting all those dormant parts of the mind into an effervescent flurry of activity. Ripples of motion were there to augment the flow of drama and eagerness. The stabs of horn and percussive attack accentuated the emotional exuberance. The acoustic avalanche was rapidly gaining momentum.

These elements were strategically positioned to focus the power that was generated from the creatively fertile ground beneath. Layers of sublime phrasing took the spirit to new and undiscovered heights. Not only did the network of tense muscularity relax, but so too did the bruised and battered psyche. Gently, but also with conviction, the essence of healing in the total sense was being delivered. Reflections and memories were put into context. All the passages hidden from conscious thought were now confronted, with the stampede of terror allowed to dissipate. As Jon and Sarah absorbed themselves in the modulating undercurrents and melodious accents, their trepidation was dissolved, with no residue left to trouble.

Now it was time for the cathedral, where everything had been received, to release all that was created to the opening of the dome. Those who had lived in self-flagellating isolation for so long would be transfixed by this spectacle, as it impressed itself upon their hearts and uplifted their withered souls. An abundance of overwhelming sensation was to be experienced when the perfect chord reached previously hidden receptors bringing about a profound mood of elevation. This assemblage of notes, all of which were perfectly executed, was present to evoke shared understanding: times when hand would be placed on hand and dreams realised. Liberty was to be strived for as the repercussions of these harmonious explorations would lead to complete blessing and release. The route to redemption was to be revealed as a method of eradicating the trials of the spirit. It was the most colossal and monumental force, an energy that was as involving as it was influential.

The orchestra punctuated the moment with the whole collective in perfect unison. The stridency of the deepest pitch of an organ's concord formed a virtual wall that offered security and protection. From the bravura of anthems to the calm of thematic refrain, all harmonic interpretation was addressed. There was a philharmonic witness evolving that promoted the ethos of reciprocal compassion. The sound of reed and brass led the ear through extremes of melodic extemporisation. There would be the reverberation of the walking bass line, underpinning a blur of animated fingers, forming smoking bebop flourishes in a manner akin to the abstract expressionists of the visual world. The tapped chordal progressions of the flamenco guitarist, highlighted by the impassioned rhythmic thump upon the wooden body, influenced the internal, intrinsic beat that governs our pattern of movement, and ultimately, life. Any aspect of discord or atmospheric cacophony was drowned out by these journeys into lands where only resolution can prosper. Jon considered his musical preparation as a foundation from which all mellifluous counterpoints can exist. Inside his surreal brain, he considered himself to be the conductor, leading and in turn defining the virtuoso touch of the lyrical, wonderful angels that made up this ethereal orchestra. Jon's ear had always been keen for he could decipher the origin and structure of complex chord sequences, as well as identify key changes and obscure time signatures. His mind was and would remain sensitive to the most subtle of nuances from which he could draw emotional depth and illuminating insight.

The polyphony was exuding the most emphatic of symphonic flourishes. The many-faceted nature of the strummed harp offered a serene and luxurious tone that combined with the rich and powerful chant of medieval plainsong. But above even those parts were the wild, untamed triplets of the soprano saxophone, which created a dreamy and reflective tonality. It wove the densest of syncopated tapestries and was also capable of bellowing and snarling like an ensnared beast. Yet this aspect of improvisation was rapidly transformed, bringing with it a mood of peaceful contemplation. This all provided the essence of a beautiful, visionary wonder that poured forth. There was strength in the swing of rhythmic motion as the roll of the kettle drum caused an expectancy that was full of impending vigour. Sections of strings and woodwind produced slices of emotive deliverance, taking all those receiving on an absorbing ride. Vast choirs only went to rescue those lost and to sacrifice their own needs as an example of benevolence. It felt as though existence was straining to be transported into the next dimension and then into eternity. The entire world was watching as these phenomena unfolded in the planetary glow above. Heavenly bodies caused all to gaze into the stars and relinquish their burdens. For now they would be laid to rest in the spirit, with each hand connected, every need offered upwards. The final reverberation would continue into the forever.

The clearly defined patterns that emanated from this synthesis were drifting into the apex, as the network of reflective images allowed the labyrinths of the inner mind to be deciphered. There was first a whirlwind of energy, overflowing and in plenitude. The decibels were rising, yet the subtleties of this dream reality remained evident. A sequence revealing differing parts was demonstrated, culminating with the revelation that all would be saved. There were symbols to be seen in the cloud bursts, as platforms of illumination were raised, but not above the dome because that was the highest point. For God was to bring the light to all.

At that moment an enormous ringing was to be heard, full of echo and protraction. This was followed by a reverberation and vibration that permeated the centre of consciousness. Every part of the mind, body and spirit, from the entry point to target, was penetrated. A roar from the beast of terror ripped through the senses as it was laid to rest and lightning struck the base of the cedar tree. There were flashes generated from electrical tension shooting down to the earth. But the trunk remained, for its strength was absolute and its gnarled bark still revealed all those years of enduring the harshest of elements. Its value to Jon and Sarah was as a perpetual symbol of sustenance to their weary souls. It was an iconic part of their lives together, lost in the glory of limitless love.

Then, in complete contrast, there was a perfect silence. Nothing could be heard as petals floated downwards from delicate branches, which hung like the graceful gesture of a principal ballerina interpreting the finest of choreographic movements. They took the form of raindrops, pouring onto the softest of green blades in profusion. The blades welcomed the drops, seeming to stretch upwards in anticipation of receiving this special fluid. The silvery moisture dripped downwards, providing refreshment and the continuation of life. In time, and as nature dictated, all the vegetation would multiply and prosper, bringing life to the previously fallow land. So the visions were symbolic and were presented to this chosen couple in complete and absolute clarity. There was no place for doubt or denial, for the message could not be challenged. So, as blossom laid down a trail on the carpet of fertile soil, a thousand tiny voices could be heard in the background. These were the children of tomorrow. The people who would carry the message onwards with commitment and zest. They had spent their time suspended in a cosmic world, preparing for the day when those who were bent over could have their sense of delight and vitality restored. There was a gentle patter of vocal rhythm directing this sense of occasion, drifting to the mountain peaks to be perceived by all. The quality of light was changing into a wondrous glow. For now there were beacons offering flames upwards, leading all paths to a new horizon.

As an all-encompassing chord was struck, the fusion was released like an uprising of the soul. The dome, which had provided a sanctuary to those without focus and the forlorn, split open, letting free all creativity. It flooded forth, like the torrents and currents of a fast-flowing river. All who witnessed this were carried away by the glistening ripples. So, as the layers of creative imagery, literature and sound had documented the trials and tribulations of a lifetime, so they expanded further and reflected the sorrow of all. The philosophy of reciprocal giving was illuminated as the perfect example to adhere to. Those images conveyed how the human being could be tried and broken and this was illustrated by posture and frozen impressions of the physical form. Just the merest suggestion of line and stroke captured that inherent fragility. Those times in the dungeons of secluded hell were documented by the tear and rip of canvas material, but this was transcended by images of complete repose, and the jewel-like quality of the forever changing light reflecting on the water's surface. From the walls of relentless confinement, swift and swallow could be seen grouped together, forming constantly altering shapes in the flame-red skies above. As Jon recalled these reassuring visions, his nib danced over the sheets of textured paper. At the start of the journey these images would adorn the enclosure that was his supposed room, but now they were visible to the tortured masses. There was now a projection of a vast, far-reaching visual diary, compiled through times of elevated mood as well as hellish depression.

This polarisation served to highlight the spectrum of experience that had gone before, and was now released. Rising above it all was the face of Christ, caught in an air of perfect contentment.

LIVES WITHIN A LIFE

The lines around his mouth bore evidence of a lightness of temperament, with all troubles resolved. This artistic outpouring was not connected to any specific religion, but rather the persistence of faith, and the fruits that can be assured when this is applied. Those who had been stripped of any dignity were now positioned to focus their intentions and step forwards. Jon had managed to capture the essence of forgiveness, from the trials of persecution, to the gift of redemption.

Words could evoke similar sensations of vulnerability, those shared perceptions of nature, the dark flaws of humanity. There were those who, in their wretched despair, would tear into their own flesh, sever arteries, even remove their gift of sight. They would lie, face down, their cranium shattered, as their disjointed minds fell apart into little pieces. A myriad of complex and terrifying disorders were evident and the prognosis was bleak. These poor persecuted individuals had to be held in rooms where there were no areas that could feasibly cause harm to them, such was their potential to carve themselves into a bloody, torn mess. Out of some strange compulsion and also because of his own experiences, Jon had immersed his thoughts in the domain of the disturbing manifestations of neurological illness.

He had endeavoured to capture this seemingly hopeless world and communicate it to those who would rather turn the other way. His love of language was prominent in his writings and he always attempted to convey detail and precision in his wordplay. These records of a troubled existence could be shared by other disorientated characters who existed on the periphery. But ultimately Jon and Sarah's dreams were to escape all of the demands that could be brought to bear on the conscious mind. Jon had considered the placing of words that formed his playful prose and spirited poems as animated characters prancing over the pages in front of weary eyes. He considered that his offerings were instrumental in the preparation of the whole release of glorification and worship. His volumes of journals containing literary expression were vital to the cause. As page after page was turned, more insight was highlighted, providing a view into the mechanics of the psyche, the chemical structures that mutate, and the derangement that inevitably ensues. Jon's inspiration was derived from the world as a whole, from its fragile beauty to the bowels of evil dislocation. The linguistic interplay was to resound internally, bringing solace and sanctuary. All of this was secure and perfectly contained.

So, as was promised, the rhythms, melodies and harmonies signified the climax of the proceedings. They instigated the release and also formed the closing of the door to darkness and derangement. The acoustics were channelled with precision, leading each individual forward whilst flooded by the light generated by the dome. Its range knew no limits, seeming to extend indefinitely. This luminosity was all-encompassing, as the common self was drenched in the warmth of beautiful and complete love. Broken hearts and broken spirits were restored and placed in a sky that poured forth a profusion of holy, pure droplets. Liberty was now tantalisingly close, for it was soon to be projected into a shared consciousness. The arrangement of notation that was inspired by an intense lifetime interpreted all of this in the form of unity for reality was now sweet and would be infused with joy.

The crescendo of celestial voices rose and intensified, yet the over riding emotion was that of peace. Here the body was held in a place of gentle tranquillity with all tension removed. From deep in the soil below, a rumble of sub bass frequencies could be felt, which was contrasted with a vocal lyricism that drifted into the mind's imagination. It was the route of the masses riding into a reconciled tomorrow. The ensuing effects were to be eternal in their impact. The percussive explosion instilled a triumphant vibrancy!

But this transference of energy conveyed a substantial movement of positive thought whilst elucidating the concept of collective compassion, where every person, whatever their state, was touched and taken away to far-away lands. They were then lifted above, beyond the atmosphere, with their pain left behind. The voices, the disturbances and the potential loss of life, were all banished by way of an explosion of cleansing, launching adversity into unreachable territories, leaving behind no residue. The conflict of aggression towards the individual, or the cruel world that surrounds all mankind, was communicated by these initially jarring chordal formations, underpinned by a twining barrage of sound. But now that had been allowed to dissolve, leaving only those ephemeral marks in the sand. The waves were soon to remove any trace of the past.

The masses were now united and everyone was smiling and full of joy, for no adversity remained as every trouble had been bound over. There was a palpable impression of expectancy, a feeling that a new and superior world was to unfold before their tired eyes. Existence was to be taken to another level, with contact made with all who had fallen before them. As the choirs harmonised, the skies revealed sparkling rays of hypnotic light, drawing attention to a retreat relative to the true definition of asylum. The vocal pitch was perfect, bringing with it exquisite exaltation and feelings of relief. These exceeded and surpassed all previous experiences. Life was now supported by layers of calm reflection and inspired exhilaration. This had brought forward the ethos of true liberty, with no more incarceration, or restriction of movement. The mind was now solid and its direction true. The monumental, gleaming bells chimed in unison.

The linear, angular beauty of the cathedral shone forth as the field of vision was directed from the base of monolithic columns to the imposing towers that crowned the vista. The gargoyles and grotesques which had symbolised the presence of the devil on this earth had now disintegrated, with only a residue of dust remaining beneath their previous position. The spires that had weathered the most brutal of onslaughts, continued to reach into the clouds above, offering a spatial suspension for the omnipotent nature of the supreme dome and its iconic status. Light radiated through complex fragments of the stained glass that adorned every annex and laid an inviting path into the heart of this place of purest worship. The Saints, angels and mere mortals were represented by way of this visual collage that captured every shade of the forever changing nature of light and its luminosity. Visions affecting the very soul were led by poetic composition and in turn were moistened by sound. The cathedral had opened its vast doors to the home of the tormented, shining its healing light as every individual passed through into the dramatic entrance. But this was only the beginning of the experience, for the pinnacle of this amazing construction was the doorway to the ultimate resting place. This was the golden, magnificent dome, where perception was to be heightened to an enlightening extreme.

The spiral path that led to the summit caused no hardship as every muscle was prepared for any effort or labour. As the chosen ones levitated, beneath them the light was extinguished, but nobody realised this for they had no temptation to look below them. They held the hand rail that guided their path, noticing, together, its smooth, tactile quality. The periphery of their sight was coloured by shades of pastel, accented by stabs of a brilliant, vivid spectrum. This visual sensation only went to reinforce their belief that they were travelling to a better place, somewhere where frailty and sensitivity would be valued and not treated with contempt and derision. They were leaving the terrors of the night, when the lost would scream into the lonely hours, trying to escape the monsters in their head. For they had been broken by the fright of bloodied demons slaughtering any innocence.

Finally, when all had entered the dome, they realised that this signified total release. Every surface was coated with shimmering gold leaf, forming curvaceous shapes that brought comfort to the withered spirits. The panelled walls were free of adornment, as there was a minimalist quality to this contained but curative environment. There were no elements of harshness, but rather a serene ambience that reached deep into the core of the resting mind. Above, the dome was constructed from glimmering glass that caught and then refracted light back down into the welcoming hall below. So, as a consequence, all present were bathed in a glorious, radiant splendour. They stood, shoulder to shoulder, gazing into the sky of intense blue, which displayed riots of star like dots and splashes, bringing about a sense of exaltation, a feeling that the revolution had begun. Their bodies started to tremble but without any fear evident. Warm, luxurious fluids coated their skin as their eyes started to close in meditative repose. Their hands clasped each other's, skin on skin. Then, out of nowhere, they felt the sensation that they were drifting upwards and, as they reopened their moistened eyes, they realised that they were floating as though suspended in a capsule without gravity. As they rose, they stroked the golden walls and caressed the columns that framed the whole internal structure. Every element was present to influence and encourage the senses to rise above, and to transcend all trials that had gone before. For now this special place was a symbol of total and complete peace.

All that remained was the metamorphosis of the tormented minds into spirit matter and for them to rise up to their final home, which offered an end to earthly pain. As motion seemed to slow down, the collective body started to turn to powder, as slithers of skin and flesh first transformed into dust and then completely evaporated into the summit of the dome. Everything was absorbed, with no traces left. Vividly kaleidoscopic birds of paradise could be seen crowning the dome, and when they looked downwards and saw that everything was complete, they opened their wings and took flight, their colouring flashing past in a variegated blur. They were joined in number, until the whole sky was full, a bold visual fantasy! They were shifting in shape, but always retained their grace and sweeping beauty. Now the people who had endured the most brutal of experiences, with most that destroyed a lifetime, were at peace, in paradise, their bodies not even left as powder.

The birds then found their final formation, rising further and further, until there was a mesmerising glow which signalled that the healing was now absolute and complete. Fullness of faith had been demonstrated, as a miracle had been performed for all the world to witness. Now, there was no more need to hurt or suffer. Those aspects of humanity were all over now, as the images, words and symphonies connected all to the same path of redemption. But the dome would remain open as all witnesses and testimonies would never be removed. Today the walls that had incarcerated were brought down to the ground and the climax had come. For all could now bathe in the residue of wonderment. It would be forever.

Jon and Sarah looked all around, aware of a definite and empowering peace. The ultimate moment had now passed, but its influence and gravity was indisputable and would never wear or erode. There was a wall of protection surrounding the dome that would never be brought down. It would never age, or be weathered by the elements and would retain its iconic beauty. As time passed by, lush and plentiful foliage was to grow over the reflecting outer walls, stretching as far as each stem could reach. The glass opening at the summit still allowed those wondrous rays to emanate, bringing about a profound, exquisite quality. The inner walls remained tall and imposing, continuing to project their strength and might. This amalgamation of sublime curve and angularity would continue to evoke feelings of warmth and relief. The dome had been the start and conclusion to a harrowing journey down sinuous paths, teetering on the edge of self-destruction. But just as every test seemed to be all-consuming, each and every individual had been caught, and carried away to safety and given infinite sanctuary. This was a place where those who were healed passed through until their final resting place in the spiritual paradise.

The dome was the symbol of all cathartic release and allowed a flood of tender light to exude, reaching the essence of every needy being that had ever existed. Pillars were directing interconnected stars which led the observers' senses to the ultimate peak: the roof of the gleaming dome. A radiant aura was left, suspended over the softest of rippling streams. Previously sedentary bodies were now animated, cavorting over fresh lawns, their eyes twinkling. There was now an answer to the question of how to balance existence. All above was now without shadow, leaving only a sea of sublime colour.

The cathedral which had harboured the elements that constituted the delivery of collective compassion stood proud. It would continue to offer a meditative refuge and a place to give thanks, for appreciation is all. This impressive, monumental building had provided the link between the worldly and secular to spiritual existence. It had been a place to discover that essence, something that reached beyond the mechanics of living and breathing. There was now a stairwell into a heavenly reality, for all those imps and demons were destroyed, as they had no remaining hold on this life. The cathedral had opened its heart to the needy, offering the route into the dome and beyond. Its foundations were absolute for there was no movement, even during those times of fiercest storm. Its spires sliced the air, their direction obvious and immediate to the troubled soul. The pure beauty of the wooden carvings and stone masonry delighted all that witnessed them.

The view from the top was glorious! But of course it was only a doorway to the ultimate promise of the dome.

As had been promised, every part and every element had been meticulously prepared, leaving the chosen pair immersed in a profound state of serenity. Their role had been both unique and precious, and they were left inside each other, entwined, their flesh bonded together. The journey was now over, the years of building and gaining provision left in the past. Now, all they could see was each other's starry eyes, their passion stronger than ever. They had truly evolved together, as the symbol of the cedar's trunk immortalised all aspects of their relationship. They had transcended the brutality of this earth, in all its extremes, and survived, emerging stronger and with their inherent vitality intact. Their blood had now become as one for they were in perfect union. There was a complete resolve and commitment to each other, with deepest roots, for they were to be always together, to be etched in time.

The faith of those chosen was to be defined through their worship. They felt a deep desire to reaffirm this belief and now the praise remained in the atmosphere and the bells would not cease ringing. The tears that had come before had poured down in abundance, cleansing any impurity and channelling it into a vast waterfall and into safety. The line and contour of the coastlines had transformed from a thing of containment into a launch pad for greater spiritual exploration. The beauty of cultural impressions would document this magnificent progression into all of the tomorrows. Jon could only imagine the scope of inspiration that could be generated by this monumental event. He then saw the image of the playful children of his early past running down the hill-sides, marks of euphoria impressed on their faces, with all trouble and concern left in the moist soil beneath. The bracken supported their every fall, for the world was now safe as an all-encompassing blanket stretched out infinitely. The days were expanding into experiences of newfound truths for the young and innocent. Dreams were now closer to the soul, the scope of creativity far-reaching. All perception was altered and had changed into attitudes of certainty and positivity. Shore-lines left only the residue of the surf as all contamination and pollution was absorbed and converted. The malediction of the vulnerable had been expelled, the curse no more. Flames were now extinguished, tears of wax severed from the stem.

Now the resolution of those who had come before was real and tangible. The air was clear, with shadows eradicated, a planet at peace. It was complete.

Out of nowhere, a view of the dome appeared supported by a dramatic cliff face. It was on the edge of a precipice, providing a vantage point to see the earth in its entirety. Jon was struggling to decipher the meaning of the monolithic symbolism. As he looked into the valley below, he experienced acute fear as he felt the compulsion to fall over into the unknown. A darker element was tempting his weaknesses to succumb. He felt his nails dig into the stone rock face, sinking ever deeper as his anxiety increased.

It was then that Sarah appeared before him, but he was unable to welcome her and she plunged over the edge. She lost control whilst accelerating, as gravity pulled her down, engulfing her slight frame. But she did not scream and all that could be seen were her eyes streaming with overflowing emotion, and eventually she left Jon's sight. His cries reached the bottom of the deepest canyon, his body bent double, his hands clasping his shivering skull. He was left to bellow into a chasm that enveloped him completely. He could not bear to lose her. Without her, he would be thrown into aching despair and crushing loneliness. There could be no way out from the sorrow, no relief from the isolation.

But, as Sarah approached the bottom of the pit, she was captured by a seraphic being and was carried away. A silver blanket broke her fall, like a woollen cushion. She was taken away and into the heavens, for she would always be protected. Jon had seen every moment of a miracle, and his heart was now full, brimming over with thanks as he fell to his knees, for he realised that the passage was complete. Every dramatic turn, every nuance, every monumental happening, all had contributed to his affection, passion and adoration for Sarah. From deep within he knew that she was the girl with evocative and intoxicating eyes. When he had looked right into them, he had been lost in a perfect world, a place where solace and benevolence were the ruling forces. Now, her eyelids never closed.

Jon was sitting, alone by the shore, looking into the ocean that reflected the gentle rippling sensations of his conscious mind. He was experiencing visions of a myriad of images, sourced from a dramatic lifetime, but nothing remained to trouble him. He playfully sifted sand through his fingers and threw the odd patterned pebble into the crashing waves existing further out. Jon felt a rhythm of steady motion from the white horses which was comforting. Footprints led a path from his location, seeming to have no end. The mountains framing the vista retained their impressive stature. Jon felt an overwhelming sense of security. He was aware that he was to be led away, and be taken to the sanctum where he would be laid to rest.

For the world he had absorbed over his years had been shattered, only to be rebuilt again as a monument to a life fantastic. He had touched and battled with hopelessness, shared the agonies of confinement and had emerged with a noble, dignified air. He had led the forlorn from the cushioned turf on the perimeter of lost asylums and taken them to paradise. From here Jon would reach into tomorrow, where the skies burst forth in a technicolor dream.

LIVES WITHIN A LIFE

CHAPTER SIX – SALVATION

On the horizon, Jon could see the peninsula, positioned on the edge of a crystalline marble landscape. The impression it made was projected upon his tranquil mood and he was drawn to its splendour. Emerging from the viewpoint, was the formation of resplendent, panoramic patterns as the setting sun's ever-expanding rays put the vile characters of yore to rest. Jon realised that great forces had been at work as the elements of mankind had been returned from fragmentation only to reveal a complete sense of belonging. Within this most splendid of images, there were brilliant displays of beauteous nature. Pea-green blades cushioned every step, providing a welcome suspension from which to direct and lead. The sound of the birds lay between the plateau of perfect contentment and the potential of infinite joy. Their song was sweet for here harmony existed and thrived. At the base of the cliffs all was harnessed that could be volatile and capricious. Jon saw that lines were etched on the stone by the shore, but now there was to be no deprivation or scarcity of compassion.

Also apparent was the provision of fruit and grain, which was there to sustain and was provided in plenitude. All that surrounded was good, and brought pleasure to the eye. The swords of burning emotion were blunted, but the vividness of passionate expression flourished. There was nothing left to languish, or to fester. The veils of deception had been dissolved as an unequivocal transformation had occurred.

This was a reality so heightened that a single vision could tell a story of a life. It was a life that had reached out beyond the ordinary and mundane, extending deep into a spiritual expedition that brought the most extraordinary insight into the human condition and the fallibility that exists within us all. To be able to survive the brutality of warfare, together with the bombardment of the soul, and then to look with the strength that exists in shared empathy. The pathways led into the distance, up until the vanishing point where they melted into the skyline. Jon realised that humanity could travel into the future, with assurance certain. The sad and the mad had been taken from those filthy, squalid corridors, their chains and shackles left by the wayside. From today, freedom was real and tangible.

Jon had now rediscovered himself and was never again to endure the pain of isolation, or the agony of desolation. He was to be wrapped and protected, his angst no more. He was living on the top of the world. And the feeling of amplitude was glorious.

There was the evidence of true advancement as the stars making up the galaxy above outlined the image of the cross. It was omnipresent and startling in its purity. Every time it was witnessed,

LIVES WITHIN A LIFE

it told the story of ultimate sacrifice and the essence of life. The ravages that these experiences had brought were now exorcised. Colossal pillars supported all that made up the kingdom. There were beacons in the atmosphere, providing sources of illumination. All the twisting streams met up in the centre of what makes up nature's rhythm. Those with sorrow in their heart could now absorb all that is bright. Every part was now in unity, overflowing with healing. For the bloodshed was no more, its droplets long gone. The light was all around, and was absolute.

Jon could feel the touch of a hand clasping his. It was warm and gentle. He paused before opening his eyes. He felt dreamy, his soul content. Every movement, though measured, was of no effort. A state of deep spiritual resolve permeated, with nothing to trouble him. Slowly, his vision revealed the source of this tactile pleasure. Beside Jon was his carer, and their eyes met in acknowledgement. They had shared much and would often spend the afternoons together, on the perfectly manicured lawns of Jon's final residence. There was a meeting of mind and spirit, leading to animated discussions, whilst above them was the sheen of golden expanse. From here Jon could follow the route of the skylarks balanced upon the edge of the towers that crowned the sanctuary. This was where he now lived with grace and elegance. All his needs were met, and he considered his life to be blessed. There was nothing now that he desired. As Jon reflected, there had been symbols of consistency in his lifetime, despite characters who had come and gone. Now here were two friends who could philosophise together, with their talk of far-reaching concepts. There was now a gentle tempo to life, a particular flow to inspire and calm.

Jon and his companion would always meet at the same bench, made to commemorate the passing of another departed soul. Daisies and buttercups crept up its rickety legs, partly preserved by flaky, discoloured paint. Above the pair were reflections of the palette of a rainbow, flashing across the sky. There was a stillness in the air, interrupted by a passing breeze that refreshed the senses. Here, within the sanctuary, there was no atmosphere of foreboding for everything was complete.

And now, here was Jon with his memories. They were so full, part of an abundant existence. Now, at the end, the key had been found. The passages, whether trials or joyous, were sealed and he had found internal salvation. An assured lucidity had evolved and nothing could now be taken away, for all the world had been given.

His companion looked deep into Jon's eyes, knowing it all. He could reach out and grab the spark of living, the drive of creation. There was no need for speech as all communication was already read. He saw all of the sadness, when the tears

LIVES WITHIN A LIFE

flowed. And the joy, when they would also flow. He heard the prayers for the disappeared, conveying the fondness for the departed. Truth now encompassed all.

Jon turned to his carer, "That was my story, my life."

"And the healing?"

"I will live on forever, with the Lord and Sarah by my side. The devil no more."

At this point his carer turned to Jon and smiled as they touched, palm to palm. He had never deserted him, carrying Jon at the times he was needed the most. For he was his guardian Angel, and now they were in a place where peace would always reign. A place called Heaven. As Jon looked above, he could see slithers of shimmering gold leaf descending from the skies. He knew that the dome would remain into eternity. They took each other by the hand and walked into the stars.

Robert Bayley

Printed in the United Kingdom
by Lightning Source UK Ltd.
135920UK00001B/76-81/P